Samyama

–

Cultivating
Stillness in Action,
Siddhis and Miracles

Yogani

From The AYP Enlightenment Series

AYP Publishing

For ordering information go to:

www.advancedyogapractices.com

Library of Congress Control Number: 2006907579

Published simultaneously in:

Nashville, Tennessee, U.S.A.
and
London, England, U.K.

This title is also available in eBook format – ISBN 0-9786496-3-X
(For Adobe Reader)

ISBN 0-9786496-2-1 (Paperback)

Life is a Miracle!

Introduction

Samyama is a powerful yoga practice that has been shrouded in mystery for centuries. Yet, it is as close to us as our immediate hopes and dreams, for it is the principles of samyama that are behind the manifestation of everything in our life.

Inner silence cultivated in deep meditation is the primary prerequisite for the *conscious* performance of samyama. With the right foundation in place, remarkable things can be achieved, including the rise of a constant flow of miracles in and around us.

The essential principles and practices of samyama are covered here, simplified in a way that enables anyone to engage in daily practice leading to results. A primary sitting samyama practice routine is provided, along with an assortment of tools that enable the practitioner to expand the applications of samyama as desired. Everyone wants something, and the use of samyama offers the possibility for us to fulfill our deepest desires.

But there is a catch. In order to fulfill our desires, we must systematically surrender them to our inner silence, to the divine within us. In doing so, all love and goodness will flow out with tremendous power. This is the way of effective samyama – whatever we surrender will come back to us a thousand-fold, and purified in a divine outpouring. This is *stillness in action...*

So, while samyama is about getting what we want, it is also about purifying and opening our nervous system to the divine within us. In doing so, our desires themselves become purified and gradually ascend to promote our highest purpose in life.

The Advanced Yoga Practices Enlightenment Series is an endeavor to present the most effective methods of spiritual practice in a series of easy-to-read books that anyone can use to gain practical results immediately and over the long term. For centuries, many of these powerful practices have been shrouded in secrecy, mainly in an effort to preserve them. Now we find ourselves in the *information age*, and able to preserve knowledge for present and future generations like never before. The question remains: "How far can we go in effectively transmitting spiritual methods in writing?"

Since its beginnings in 2003, the writings of *Advanced Yoga Practices* have been an experiment to see just how much can be conveyed, with much more detail included on practices than in the spiritual writings of the past. Can books provide us the specific means necessary to tread the path to enlightenment, or do we have to surrender at the feet of a *guru* to find our salvation? Well, clearly we must surrender to something, even if it is to our own innate potential to live a freer and happier life. If we are able to do that, and maintain regular practice, then books like this one can come alive and instruct us in the ways of human spiritual transformation. If the reader is ready and the book is worthy, amazing things can happen.

While one person's name is given as the author of this book, it is actually a distillation of the efforts of thousands of practitioners over thousands of years. This is one person's attempt to simplify and make practical the spiritual methods that many have demonstrated throughout history. All who have gone before have my deepest gratitude, as do the many I am privileged to be in touch with in the present who continue to practice with dedication and good results.

I hope you will find this book to be a useful resource as you travel along your chosen path.

Practice wisely, and enjoy!

Table of Contents

Chapter 1 – The Making of Miracles

What determines achievement? Is it getting what we want, or is it giving up what we want? Interestingly, it is both, and not necessarily in that order. There is a natural process of gaining knowledge and its associated achievements that has been observed in human beings since the beginning of our history. To understand it is to know the secret of making miracles.

We have all known people of achievement. No doubt we ourselves have accomplished things in this life, and no doubt would like to achieve more. There is the old adage that success is achieved by staying focused on our chosen task. Persistent hard work toward our goal is the prescribed formula we have heard since childhood.

Yet, why is it that great innovators like Sir Isaac Newton and Albert Einstein tell us that they made their greatest discoveries while doing absolutely nothing? Why is it that artists tell us that their most beautiful creations flow through them, with the main work being to keep up with that outflow?

Is there something systematic and effortless we can do that will greatly enrich our endeavors in everyday life? We will explore it here, and present an age-old method of yoga called *samyama* that takes advantage of a principle in us that can give rise to remarkable achievements, even entering the realm of the miraculous, all coming from within as a natural flow of energy and creativity.

The samyama methods we will be discussing here are easy and practical, and can help us make good use of the vast resources that are available within us right now.

How Our World is Manifested

It says in the *Bible* that, "In the beginning was the word…"

And before that, what was there? Stillness, nothingness – an infinite field of potential.

Then along came a vibration from the void – a word. An intention, we could say. And from that, "…all things were made."

In other words, the creation of the physical universe came out of a vibration occurring in stillness, coming out of emptiness. Talk about making something out of nothing. For lack of a better explanation, astronomers call it "the big bang."

With all of this going on, what has happened to that stillness, that infinite field of potential? Absolutely nothing. It is still with us, comfortably resting beneath the creation that came from it. It is the eternal reality behind the mask of the material universe, and our world.

In the field of physics, this has been recognized quite clearly. We now know that what seems to be solid is in every respect nothing but empty space with miniscule points of energy whirling around each other through the emptiness, giving the *appearance and sensation* of physical matter. Physicality is a product of our perception. This appearance and sensation of the physical is very real, as we all have found out when we have banged into some of that empty physical matter. Yet, we know that it is empty, all the same. Strange, isn't it?

So, even though we seem to have a rather frail and vulnerable existence here on the physical plane, we know there is more to it than that. There is a dynamic involved in all of this that comes from stillness, from emptiness, from eternity. Not only that, we know that there is a great intelligence involved. Can we look at a rose, a butterfly, or any living thing, and say there is no intelligence coming out into expression on this physical plane? To deny an innate intelligence is to deny the obvious. Surely there is a vast intelligence expressing itself everywhere we look. And it comes from within, constantly manifesting from emptiness. Life is truly a miracle!

Einstein said that we can consider everything to be a miracle, or nothing. It makes no sense to be picking and choosing our miracles from this vast and wondrous universe. Either it all is a miracle or none of it is. The Buddha said that if we could see the miracle in a single flower, our view of everything would change. In layman's terms, perhaps a miracle is that which we have not yet taken for granted. Once we fully wake up to the reality around us, nothing is taken for granted anymore.

And so it is with human beings too. We are part of the miracle of life, that endless intelligence bubbling out from stillness into material expression. Obviously, not everyone is in tune with this fundamental truth. We do tend to get a bit distracted from our roots, and enmeshed in materiality. The more enmeshed we become, the less innate intelligence we have access to, and the less we are able to accomplish what we want in this world. Life becomes a struggle when we can no longer operate from our source, from our center.

If we wish to achieve our goals with maximum creative expression, and with less effort, the obvious answer is to get in touch with the source of all creativity and intelligence, the source that can be found in the stillness within us. This is accomplished by untangling our silent inner awareness from the habitual attachments we have developed that have limited our expression on this earth. This untangling is a process of inner *purification and opening*. There are highly effective, time-tested ways for accomplishing this, ways that put us in alignment with the vast forces within us that have created the entire universe. It is through our own mind, emotions, body and nervous system that the connection is achieved. Our possibilities for expression are as unlimited as the infinite field of potential that underlies everything. We only need to learn how to tap into it.

Discovering Our Vast Inner Potential

There are layers that constitute our physical and non-physical existence. The methods of *yoga* are geared toward activating the principles of evolution within us that unify our awareness and functioning throughout these layers. Before we have undertaken the practices of yoga, we may only be aware of the external layers of our existence via the senses, intellect and emotions. It is a limited view, with corresponding limits in our ability to fulfill our desires. It turns out that we can use these same aspects of our nature to go much deeper.

Yoga means *to join,* or *union*. Hence, the methods of yoga are for fully joining our inner and outer nature. In doing that, many new revelations and capabilities will come to us. It is a homecoming, a discovery of our full potential, which has been there within us all the time.

But where should we start on our quest to tap our full potential? It is a complex undertaking. Fortunately, the means can be greatly simplified so anyone can immediately begin to open inwardly to great peace, knowledge and power, and continue to expand on these innate qualities throughout life. The possibilities are very exciting.

The essential constituent in all of this is the cultivation of inner silence, which is accomplished first through daily deep meditation practice. This is where it begins. It is not so much to do – sitting for a few minutes morning and evening with an easy and powerful mental procedure. Once we have some inner silence coming up and stabilizing in our nervous system, many other possibilities open to us, including the practice of samyama.

Inner silence has many other names – stillness, the witness, yoga nidra, samadhi, pure bliss consciousness, sat-chit-ananda, tao, void, emptiness, infinite intelligence, transcendence, and so on. They all mean the same, with varying points of emphasis – describing that inner silence which all human beings are capable of cultivating and sustaining naturally. In the Bible it is written, "Be still, and know that I am God." Similar injunctions can be found in many of the ancient scriptures of the world.

Humanity has been aware of its potential for a long time, if not the means to cultivate it reliably. Now that is changing in these times of rising knowledge and more effective applications of the principles of human spiritual transformation that reside within all of us.

So we begin with deep meditation, which is covered in detail in the AYP writings. Twice each day for 20 minutes or so, every day, like clockwork, and our inner silence begins to stir in us. But wait a minute. How can silence stir? How can stillness move?

This is one of the great mysteries of spiritual growth – the awakening of infinite immovable silence within us. And it is moving! It is a miracle of the human nervous system, an incredible vehicle of life that can contain and dynamically express that which is both infinite and immovable. But is it such a miracle? Look around you right now. Everything you see is an expression of that same infinite and immovable presence. We don't have to go far to find a miracle. We are the miracle, and it is all around us in everything we see in every moment. The more integrated we become from the outside in and the inside out through effective yoga practices, the more obvious it becomes.

Besides *inner silence*, there is another element of our inner unfoldment that is good to understand before we charge ahead into the methods of samyama. It is the rise of *ecstatic conductivity* within us, which is the movement of ecstatic energy throughout our nervous system. The Sanskrit word for energy is *prana*, which is stillness (pure bliss consciousness) moving to manifest and animate all of material existence, including our inner neurobiological functioning.

Ecstatic conductivity is an ever-increasing flow of energy/prana, and is the means by which stillness moves within us, and far beyond. It is also the means by which our sensory perception becomes highly refined. Both inner silence and ecstatic conductivity are cultivated in deep meditation. The rise of ecstatic conductivity is greatly enhanced through additional specialized practices involving the breath, body and sexuality. In the AYP writings many techniques are provided in addition to deep meditation, with one of the most important being spinal breathing pranayama.

With a balanced twice-daily practice of deep meditation and spinal breathing pranayama, we are cultivating both inner silence and ecstatic conductivity. Together, these provide the fertile ground for the movement of inner silence through us, and outward. This is both the discovery of our inner potential, and the cultivation of it for our benefit and the benefit of others. To put it in more glamorous terms, we can also call it the rise of abiding pure bliss consciousness, ecstatic bliss, and outpouring divine love.

Whatever we choose to call the process, it is quite attainable by anyone. As we engage in our practices, every step of development along the way is a new beginning of possibilities for greater joy and fulfillment that we could not imagine before. It is the stuff of miracles, and it is here with us right now, ready for the asking.

Becoming a Channel of Infinite Expression

Some may be reading here who are interested in developing siddhis (yogic powers), becoming a healer, or miracle maker. Or maybe there are some gifts present already and we would like to expand on them. This is fine, but it is a fact that none of us will reach our full potential as long as we are only projecting our awareness outward into the thing we are seeking. Neither can we be as successful or fulfilled as we would like by attempting to possess an external expression of power. It just does not work that way.

Real spiritual power cannot be owned or applied for our personal use. It is much better than that.

<u>Real spiritual power is essentially what we are, and it flows through us effortlessly as we attune ourselves to our own inner nature</u>.

It might seem strange to say that what we already are we cannot own for our personal use. The truth is that we own it as we become our *Self*, our inner silence. Before then we are merely banging on the gate. It is foolhardy to be demanding what is in the castle from outside before we have taken up residence in the castle that has been ours all along. As it says in the Bible, "Seek first the kingdom of heaven, and all will be added to you." It is important to understand this point. If we want the treasure, we have to claim the castle that contains the treasure. In doing that, our entire life and point of view will be expanded in glorious ways, and the treasure will be lying around everywhere. We might not even notice the treasure because living in the castle is so much better than having the treasure. The treasure we thought would be so wonderful is a mere bauble compared to life in the castle. One thing is for sure. We will never get the castle or the treasure by chasing the treasure alone. On the other hand, we will always get the treasure if we take up permanent residence in the castle. Is this such a difficult choice to make?

So, if this is the case, why bother with the treasure at all? Many make this argument, speaking of yogic powers and such like they are the problem, a plague to be avoided at all costs. Well, it seems logical, except for one thing. In order to advance toward enlightenment (move into our castle), it is necessary to fully purify and open our nervous system to our inner reality and capabilities.

The purification and opening of the nervous system is a rather large project for most of us, and we need every tool at our disposal to progress as quickly as possible with the work. As we will see in the next chapter, the real genius of yoga is in the multiple angles (limbs) it has available for this work, with samyama being the icing on the cake of yoga, so to speak.

The practice of samyama is therefore not for the development of powers, but for advancing the process of purification and opening within us. Put another way, there is so much treasure lying around the doorway leading into the castle that we literally have to wade through the treasure to enter the castle. It is not such a tricky business if we come to samyama with a good foundation of inner silence, which means a good foundation in deep meditation. Without inner silence we will not even find the doorway to the castle, or any treasure either – inner silence is the doorway, the castle, the treasure, and everything else.

But this is a bit of an oversimplification, because with our daily practices over months, years and decades, our inner purification and opening goes on, and on, and on, reaching ever more celestial heights. It simply does not end. Indeed, enlightenment is not as much a final destination as it is a never-ending journey of increasing divine expression. It is happening all around us in nature, yes? And we can continue the process as our individual evolution expands to become the evolution of our community, nation, world and the entire cosmos. As we become established in our inner silence and then begin moving outward through it ecstatically, we literally become a channel of infinite expression in the world. This is not a personal mission we carve out for ourselves. It is the natural expression of what we are as we continue to engage in our practices and go out into daily activity in a very normal way. There is nothing so exotic about it. It is only life being lived as it can be lived, in joy, freedom and outpouring divine love.

Samyama is an essential ingredient in all of this, because it stimulates the movement of pure bliss consciousness (our inner silence) to flow outward into expression in the world.

This is why samyama is so often associated with siddhis and miracles. But the siddhis and miracles are incidental to the much greater process that is going on. If we want siddhis and miracles for ourselves, we cannot have them, not without incurring a large cost to our evolution (the dark side). But if we want to help others and take care of our inner business (the cultivation of inner silence and ecstatic conductivity), we will constantly be surrounded by spontaneous miracles, in addition to the sea of miracles we are living in already.

The real blessing is not the miracles themselves, but the fact that we human beings have the ability to fully express the infinite divine intelligence that resides within us.

Now that we have covered a few of the basics, let's move into the practice of samyama. As we go along, we will expand on the possibilities mentioned so far. What we will find is that we are dealing with a universal principle that is found in many fields of human endeavor. It is the business of learning how to manifest the very best we have to offer from within ourselves. We have much more to give than we ever imagined, and we can do it with relative ease.

By the time we are done here, we will have covered a formidable array of samyama tools that can be used in practical ways to enhance our life and the lives of our loved ones, friends and everyone else both near and far.

Chapter 2 – Samyama

While yoga is a fascinating subject to read about, ponder and discuss, the real benefits come from practice. By this we do not mean an occasional dipping in of the toe, though that is better than nothing. What we mean is daily practice over months and years. If we do that with some dedication, we can experience huge improvements in the quality of our life.

It isn't so difficult. We are not talking about going off to live in a cave or anything like that. As a matter of fact, with an efficient approach to yoga practices, like we discuss in the AYP writings, it can all be done in a half-hour, more or less, twice each day. So we can continue with our regular daily life as we did before. As a matter of fact, it is preferred that we continue with life as before, because this helps stabilize what we gain in our daily practices, and this speeds our progress along the road toward enlightenment.

We will find that samyama is an optimized approach to doing what we have been doing for all our life already – moving toward what we want. With a difference. We will learn to systematically *let go* of what we want, and in doing so, we will receive it a thousand-fold. The principle of samyama is the same one found in the sometimes popular and always perennial methods for utilizing our innate ability to attract what we want into our life (*law of attraction, law of abundance*, etc.). In doing so, we are releasing the things that have been holding us back. Samyama is a systematic and highly efficient way of doing this. It can work for everyone, because everyone is endowed with a human nervous system. It is the human nervous system that is the doorway to the infinite, and to all that flows from that divine realm within us.

Let's take a quick look at where the knowledge of samyama comes from, so we will have an understanding of its context within the overall scheme of yoga. No part of yoga stands alone. Each practice we find in yoga is a part of the whole, and the whole of yoga is much greater than the sum of its parts.

The Yoga Sutras of Patanjali

Samyama is a word that we find in an ancient Indian scripture called the *Yoga Sutras of Patanjali*. It is one of the greatest scriptures of all time, because it codifies in a few pages the essential principles and practices for cultivating the natural process of human spiritual transformation. All scriptures contain elements of the famous eight limbs of yoga described in the *Yoga Sutras*. But very few scriptures contain all of the limbs. So, besides being an excellent guide on the essentials of spiritual practice, the *Yoga Sutras* make a pretty good checklist by which the efficacy of any spiritual path can be measured.

The eight limbs of yoga are simple to list:

Yama: Restraints – non-violence, truthfulness, non-stealing, preservation and cultivation of sexual energy, and non-covetousness.

Niyama: Observances – purity/cleanliness, contentment, focus/intensity, spiritual/self study, and surrender to our highest ideal.

Asana: Those yoga postures we all know and love.

Pranayama: Breathing techniques for awakening and cultivating the inner ecstatic energies.

Pratyahara: Introversion of sensory perception – awakening to inner space and beyond, ultimately transcending sensory attachments altogether.

Dharana: Putting attention on an object.

Dhyana: Meditation – natural dissolving of the object in the mind.

Samadhi: Absorption of the object and attention in stillness, inner silence, pure bliss consciousness.

Samyama is a specific means for combining the last three of the eight limbs of yoga to produce a natural flow of inner silence outward, or what we call *stillness in action*.

While the limbs of yoga are fairly easy to list and ponder, practice is another matter. The most difficult part of yoga practice is keeping it simple!

There is a common tendency among yoga practitioners to take a rigid and difficult approach to the eight limbs of yoga. This can happen easily if one starts at the beginning with the restraints and observances, focusing on perfecting those before being permitted to move on to the more powerful practices further down the list. In this case, we can end up with a life lived by rules of conduct, with the natural joy and spontaneity of the inner divine life being somewhat hard to come by.

This is not the approach in the AYP writings. Instead, we go through the list somewhat backwards, and find the beginning of the list so much more natural and easy that way, manifesting on its own from inner silence, with rigid enforcement of the rules of conduct rarely being necessary. We find the divine qualities of harmonious conduct coming from within us automatically.

We do this by beginning with deep meditation, and then a form of pranayama we call spinal breathing. Besides making for an easy and enjoyable approach to the eight limbs of yoga, beginning in this way fulfills a very important prerequisite for samyama. As was mentioned in the last chapter, if we do not have resident inner silence, samyama practice will not be doing much. So this is the route that is suggested. It is quick and effective, and brings much peace and joy right from the start. Then we will find all of our practices coming along very well, including samyama. Before we know it, we will be noticing the rise of inner silence in our daily life (the witness), and divine energy pouring out in everything we do.

The Technique of Samyama

Deep meditation is the process of easily bringing the attention inward to stillness, inner silence, pure bliss consciousness, the witness state, samadhi. All of these are describing the same thing. We have a particular deep meditation procedure that we do for a set amount of time twice-daily. The procedure of deep meditation is fully covered in *Deep Meditation – Pathway to Personal Freedom*, and in the *AYP Easy Lessons* book.

Deep meditation works like clockwork and, over time, as we meditate each day and then go out and are active, our nervous system becomes naturally accustomed to sustaining and radiating inner silence. Our daily life then becomes calmer from the inside. We are less overwhelmed by external events. This is the rise of the first stage of enlightenment, which is inner silence present in our life, twenty-four hours per day, seven days per week (24/7).

Once we have some abiding inner silence, even just a little, we have the opportunity to begin to operate from that level of infinite potential residing within us. All that exists is manifested from that, and we, being that, are capable of manifesting from that infinite reservoir of life within us. So, with our toe in infinite inner silence, we can begin to move from there for the benefit of our purification and opening toward enlightenment. It is simple to do.

In deep meditation we use the thought of a sound, a mantra, to systematically allow the mind to go to stillness. In the case of using a mantra we do not use meaning, language or intellectual content, even if our mantra happens to have a meaning in a particular language. We just easily pick up the mental sound of the mantra, and we are able to dive deep into pure bliss consciousness. The nervous system also goes to silence with the mind, and our metabolism slows way down.

With samyama, we go the other way, from the inside out, instead of from the outside in. And we use meaning.

After our deep meditation time is up, we sit quietly for a minute or two, and then we transition into samyama. We begin, continuing in our customary sitting position with eyes closed, in an easy state of not minding any mental activity, just resting in our silence. If thoughts are coming, we just let them go without entertaining them. In samyama practice we do not entertain our mantra either. We start by not favoring anything but being easy in our silence, however much silence we have from our just completed meditation session, and also naturally present in us from our months or years of daily deep meditation. This is the starting point for samyama – abiding inner silence, stillness.

The only prerequisite for doing samyama practice is having some inner silence. For most people this is after a few months of daily deep meditation. The rise of ecstatic conductivity, cultivated with spinal breathing pranayama and other means, is a great help in samyama also, but is not a primary prerequisite for samyama practice. Ecstatic conductivity plays a key role in providing a medium for transmission of the *effects* of samyama. This will be discussed a little later. For getting started with samyama, abiding inner silence, cultivated in deep meditation, is the key.

Maybe we have been doing another kind of meditation, or are just naturally quiet inside. Will samyama work for us? Maybe. There is only one way to find out. Try and see. Do keep in mind that our samyama practice will be most successful if we have a reliable daily meditation practice that will continue to cultivate abiding inner silence in us. The two practices work together like that. Remember what we said about the whole of yoga being more than the sum of the parts.

Samyama Technique Explained

With samyama, we are initiating meaning in inner silence. We do it in a simple, easy, systematic way. First we create an impulse of meaning in silence using a specific word or short phrase, and then we let it go in silence.

Let's begin with *Love*. It is a good place to start with samyama. In samyama it is suggested you use your most intimate language, the language that goes deepest in your heart, whatever it may be. So, unlike with mantra, samyama words can be translated to another language.

In your easy silence, pick up, just once, the fuzziest feeling of the word *Love*. Don't deliberately make a clear pronunciation, or mental images of this or that scene or situation that represent *Love* to you. Just have a faint remembrance of the word *Love*, and then let it go into your silence, the easy silence you are in as you pick up the faint word *Love*. Don't contemplate *Love* or analyze it during samyama. Contemplation is an impediment to samyama. So don't think about it at all.

We don't make an effort to physically locate the word *Love* in the body. If it is here or there in a physical location, we don't mind. We don't locate it, or try to stop it from being in a location.

Just come to the word *Love* once in a faint, subtle way, and then let it go into silence. It is a subtle feeling of the word *Love* we are coming to, nothing more, and letting then it go. Like that.

Having thought *Love* once, be in silence for about 15 seconds. If any thoughts come, let them go easily. Don't try and push thoughts out, or hang onto them. Be neutral about whatever happens after picking up and letting go of the word.

We do not deliberately coordinate our samyama with breathing, or any other internal or external phenomena.

It is not necessary to look at the clock to measure the 15 seconds. With a little practice your inner clock will tell you with good enough accuracy when 15 seconds are up. Just be easy in silence for about a quarter of a minute. Then pick up the faint, fuzzy word *Love* again, and let it go into your silence for about 15 seconds again.

That is two repetitions of samyama – twice picking up *Love* at its subtlest level of thought, and twice letting it go into inner silence.

What is the effect of this? What will happen?

To the extent we are picking up the word on the faint and fuzzy border of inner silence (the subtlest level of thought), and then letting go easily into stillness, the effect will be very powerful. Inner silence is a huge amplifier of subtle thought. As a matter of fact, inner silence is the only amplifier of thought. It is the wellspring of thought. Usually our thoughts come out of silence colored by all that is lodged in our subconscious mind. So many habitual patterns are lodged in our obstructed subconscious mind, and these are what distort and weaken the flow of divine energy coming out from inner silence into our everyday life. With meditation we are clearing out the obstructions in the subconscious mind and developing a clear presence of our inner silence. With samyama we are acting directly within our inner silence to produce a powerful outflow of positive effects that purify our nervous system and surroundings.

During samyama we may feel some energy moving out from our silence. It can be experienced as physical, mental or emotional. Or maybe we won't feel much until later on in our daily activity, and then we may be more loving and compassionate for no obvious external reason. We are changing from the inside. This is what samyama is – moving our own intentions from the divine level of silence in us outward into external manifestation. In doing so, our thoughts become purified to a higher purpose, and are greatly strengthened.

No matter what thought we use in samyama, the effect will be purification and opening with great power. Real samyama *always* produces a positive outcome, no matter what we release into our inner silence. This is a vital point that is little understood. Understanding this and verifying it in our own experience dispels the fear, superstition and dire warnings that often surround the subject of samyama. Such warnings and fears are unfounded. Samyama is about purifying and opening all that is within us, including *any thought* we can conceive of, no matter how negative. Inner silence will transform the most negative thoughts (obstructions) into a river of divine love. We will make practical use of this principle in the next chapter.

The only negative effects we may experience in samyama may come from overdoing in practice, which can lead to excess energy flows associated with purification and opening. In other words, too much of a good thing. We will cover effective measures for dealing with such occurrences (see *self-pacing*). When choosing words to use in samyama, our main objective is to have a balanced over all approach to purification and opening, rather than focusing on this or that individual word or phrase.

Samyama is what prayer is when taken to its deepest level of communion within us, and released within divine inner silence. As we will see in the next chapter, effective prayer is based on the principles of samyama, and can involve just about any quality or obstacle we would like to illuminate with pure bliss consciousness from within, assuming we have met the prerequisite of having some abiding inner silence.

Sutras for Balanced Purification and Opening

Each word or phrase we use in samyama is called a *sutra*. In Sanskrit, sutra means, *tied together*, or *stitched*. The English medical word, *suture* comes from *sutra*. When used in samyama, sutras are *code words* or *phrases* that represent particular meanings. We use sutras to telegraph particular meanings into unbounded pure bliss consciousness. There they are purified and amplified out through us into everyday life. This process *joins* our inner and outer life. So, sutras are aspects of yoga (union) we can consciously cultivate in ourselves through samyama practice. Taken together, a well-selected list of sutras can provide broad-based purification in our nervous system, and far beyond.

As with all yoga practices, the benefits from samyama are to be found in long term daily practice. If we use a balanced routine of sutras and practice regularly, great benefits will accumulate gradually in our life. If we keep changing sutras around every day or week, and are irregular in our practice, the results will be diluted accordingly.

If we want to strike water, we will do best to keep digging in the same place. We can do samyama after every meditation session, and then take 5-10 minutes of rest at the end. Samyama is a continuation of our sitting practice, which includes spinal breathing pranayama followed by deep meditation. With pranayama and meditation, we are going in, and then we are coming out with samyama. So, once we have completed our deep meditation, we relax in silence for a minute or two on our seat, and then begin samyama.

For our samyama practice, a balanced series of nine sutras are given here, covering a full range of qualities, which will provide for balanced purification and opening in our nervous system. The suggestion is for each sutra to be done for two cycles of samyama, picking up each faintly two times with about 15 seconds in silence for each repetition, and going through the list in order like that. In a few days they will be memorized and easy to navigate through using this method of samyama, going gradually deeper in practice with each session.

The sutras are:

- **Love**

- **Radiance**

- **Unity**

- **Health**

- **Strength**

- **Abundance**

- **Wisdom**

- **Inner Sensuality**

- **Akasha – Lightness of Air**

Each sutra is to be picked up faintly in its entirety, and released with about 15 seconds in silence afterward, using the same technique we described for *Love*.

For example, *Inner Sensuality* is a single sutra followed by 15 seconds of silence. This sutra is for *pratyahara* (introversion of the senses). *Akasha – Lightness of Air* is also a single sutra, followed by fifteen seconds in silence. It is to promote lightness of body, and the corresponding lightness of heart and mind.

As mentioned earlier, the sutras can be translated to our most familiar language. In the case of *Akasha*, this is a Sanskrit word meaning *inner space*. The words *Inner Space – Lightness of Air* can be translated to create the sutra in another language, if desired. We know from physics that we are empty space inside, nothing really solid in here at all. Our body is that, and when we do samyama on *Akasha – Lightness of Air*, or its equivalent, *Inner Space – Lightness of Air* we begin to feel very spacious and light. When we know the body is empty space, it can be easily transported anywhere.

If you do each of these nine sutras twice in your samyama session, letting go each time for 15 seconds, it will take about five minutes. If there is a particular sutra you feel the need to do more of, then add that one to the end and do samyama with it exclusively for another five minutes. The cycles remain at 15 seconds with the last sutra, and we just keep going with that for the additional five minutes. There is no need to count repetitions during the last five minutes of practice. We can just peek at the clock when about five minutes have passed. When time is up, then stop and rest for 5-10 minutes. If there is room to lie down during rest, this is good. Otherwise, just lean back comfortably during the rest period.

If there is no preference, then you can use the lightness sutra for five minutes at the end. It is very powerful. It is a mental technique that brings much energy up through the nervous system. It is not uncommon to experience physical symptoms such as panting (a form of automatic pranayama), shaking and hopping during samyama with the lightness sutra. If this happens, make sure you are sitting on a soft surface like a mattress. There can be a variety of symptoms manifesting with the other sutras as well.

We are moving infinite inner silence from within us, so the manifestations coming out can be very real and noticeable. Patanjali calls these manifestations *super-normal powers*, or *siddhis*. Our energy surges and physical symptoms represent the early stages of siddhis. Later on, as inner purification and opening advance, the physical symptoms we may have experienced will become much less, and we will notice spontaneous events in our life signifying inner support rising all around us. This is the natural rise of siddhis and miracles in our everyday life as we are purified and opened from within.

The symptoms we may experience beforehand are the result of energy encountering inner obstructions in our nervous system. The sensations and movements are caused by *friction* as our inner energies are gradually dissolving the obstructions. As the nervous system becomes purified, the friction becomes less, even as the energy flow increases to bring increasingly wonderful manifestations of divine grace into our daily life.

Whatever the symptoms may be, we just easily favor the simple procedure of our samyama. We do not favor thought streams, energy movements, physical movements, breathing patterns, or any other symptoms that may come up during samyama. We don't try and force our experience one way or the other. We just favor the easy procedure of samyama, and the rest comes naturally.

Moral Self-Regulation

In the third chapter of the *Yoga Sutras of Patanjali* on *Super-Normal Powers*, a variety of sutras are given. They are reviewed in the Appendix of this book from a practical point of view. The sutras are offered in simplified form, so research on them may be undertaken, if desired, once we have become well established in our daily routine of samyama practice as presented in this chapter and the next one. Research using an open list of sutras, as may be derived from those offered by Patanjali, is not recommended before then. This is further discussed in the Appendix.

All that we are presenting on samyama and sutras is not for obtaining instant results or powers. If it were, we would not be doing any favors in terms of helping anyone advance along the road to enlightenment. As pointed out by Patanjali, powers for their own sake would be great distraction to yoga, if they were so easily obtained on the level of limited ego consciousness.

Fortunately, samyama is a *morally self-regulating* practice, which means inner silence (samadhi) is the prerequisite for success in samyama. Inner silence is beyond ego consciousness. If there is inner silence, there will also be rising moral responsibility and conduct (yama and niyama), due to the natural connectedness of all the limbs of yoga. Along with this comes dispassion for the external performances of siddhis. Interestingly, the more advanced we become in our samyama practice, the less attachment we will have to the results. The flip side of this is that the more interested we are in siddhis, the less effective our samyama will be, because we will have less inner silence. This is *self-regulation* coming from within.

So, the dire warnings we so often hear about powers derived from samyama are overstated. Whatever sort of attachments we are warned about cannot come from effective samyama practice, because effective samyama practice is without attachments (beyond ego), by definition.

Samyama is having inner silence (samadhi), the ability to pick up a thought (focus/dharana), and let it go inward (meditation/dhyana), all at the same time. Then the results of samyama come out from inner silence automatically. If we have the last three limbs of yoga (samyama), we will also have all the other limbs of yoga manifesting (they are all connected within us), so any powers arising from samyama will be divine in purpose.

Even so, we should be clear about our experiences versus our practices, and be mindful not to get too caught up in experiences that come up. Whenever experiences do come up, we easily come back to the practice we are doing. This is important, because experiences do not produce spiritual progress. Practices do. So, while there is not any great risk of calamity within samyama practice, the experiences we will encounter sooner or later can distract us, and water down our practice. This can happen if we go off the procedure of our practice and engage ourselves in the *scenery*, as it were. This is why we easily favor our practices over our experiences in all aspects of our yoga routine, not only in samyama. When we are out of practices in our daily activity, we can indulge in our inner experiences and enjoy them if we wish. There will be plenty to enjoy!

Let's make sure to take plenty of rest when coming out of our routine of practices, especially when doing samyama. Lying down for 5-10 minutes at the end is ideal – longer is okay too. Mental techniques such as deep meditation and samyama are very powerful. They produce a lot of purification and opening within us, so it is important to rest at the end of our sitting routine to allow everything to settle down inside. It is equally important to go out into activity after our practices and rest. Full engagement in activity in our daily life will stabilize what we have gained in our practices, and produce permanent positive effects.

It is important not to overdo in our practices, as this can result in uncomfortable energy flows during and after practices. Later in this chapter, we will discuss application of the principles of *self-pacing*, which will enable us to maintain maximum progress with comfort and safety.

Samyama greatly strengthens our presence in the silence of pure bliss consciousness. It promotes an integration of the inner and outer aspects of our neurobiological functioning. It stimulates the nervous system to purify and open, leading to a continuous flow of silent bliss outward from within us.

We call it *stillness in action*, making the overall power of our desires much stronger. When we want to accomplish something that is in tune with the divine flow, resistance will be much less and obstacles will seem to melt away. If our initial desires are misguided, they will be redirected from within in ways that invariably lead to a positive outcome. For those who live in the silence of pure bliss consciousness and develop the habit of functioning naturally from that infinite level of life, a constant stream of *small miracles* becomes commonplace.

None of this has to be taken on faith. Try samyama practice for a few months after your twice-daily deep meditation practice, and see for yourself. Samyama is much more than a sitting practice. It is a means for culturing thinking and doing in our everyday life in a way that brings out the higher purpose that resides within us. As this occurs, we are naturally propelled along our path toward enlightenment.

Questions and Answers on Daily Practice

As soon as we begin our daily practice of samyama, questions are bound to come up. They can be on subjects ranging from the basics of the technique to new experiences that can occur. We will cover some of the key questions on practice here, and delve into the dynamics of experiences in the following sections.

Nothing much seems to be happening during samyama. Am I ready for this?
You are ready if you sense some abiding inner silence, feel in your heart you are ready, and if you can sustain a daily practice. As with deep meditation, we do not measure the results of samyama by what is happening during the practice itself. The real measure will be in how we feel during our daily activities, in-between our sittings. If we feel more peace, creativity and happiness in life, that will be a good indication of results occurring, even if our samyama sittings are uneventful. This is true of all yoga practices.

The fruit of yoga is found not in what happens during the practices themselves, but in how they affect the quality of our life.

What is the difference between picking up and releasing the word, Love, and contemplating Love during samyama?
The sutras we use in samyama are code words for information that is already embedded deep within us with language. Picking up the sutra alone and releasing it into our inner silence will merge the full content of meaning automatically with our resident pure bliss consciousness, just as speaking a word out loud will automatically convey its meaning externally to anyone who understands our language. If we understand our language, so does our inner silence, so we need not worry about conveying meaning with our sutras.

We do not *contemplate* during samyama, as this will keep us engaged in thinking and prevent the absorption of the sutra in inner silence. Less is more when we are going inward. We just follow the easy procedure for picking up the sutra at that very faint and fuzzy level every 15 seconds, and let it go. Very simple.

If we wish to contemplate the meaning of our sutras outside samyama practice, this is fine. It is good for us to understand the meaning and intent of our sutras. It is we who determine that. It does not come from somewhere else. It will become part of our inner programming, as is the case with all language. This is why we do the sutras in our own language, so the meaning of the words will be alive in seed form deep within us. It is not necessary to overdo it and think about the meaning of our sutras all day. We just easily come to know what they are and what they mean. That's all. When we sit to do samyama, we forget all that and just use the sutras as suggested, and the best results will be there.

There is a story in the Bible about how difficult it is for a rich man to enter the kingdom of heaven, as difficult as a camel going through the eye of a needle. It is like that with samyama too. If we are "rich" with thinking and meanings, contemplation, etc. during our samyama, then letting go into inner silence will be like trying to put a camel through the eye of a needle – nearly impossible. But if we pick up the sutra in that very faint and fuzzy way in the mind and let it go, then it will go into inner silence easily. The camel will become very small and indistinct, almost nothing at all, and go right through the eye of the needle. Then the results will be very good. That is how samyama works.

I am having trouble keeping with the 15-second interval. Any suggestions? And why 15 seconds?

In samyama, timing is simply a matter of developing a habit. It takes several sittings to do that. The nervous system actually has a very accurate clock built into it, and we can access it simply by engaging it repeatedly in our practice. In deep meditation this is true, and it is true in samyama also. However, there is a difference.

In deep meditation, most of us will follow the easy procedure for 20 minutes. Peeking at the clock near the end of the session is a suitable way of confirming where we are in time.

In samyama, we don't want to be peeking at the clock to verify every 15-second interval. That would be too much distraction from the natural process we are engaged in. Instead, what we do is go through all of our sutras for the two repetitions each and check our time near the end, or when we are done. Then we will know if we have been going too fast or too slow, and we can make an adjustment the next time we sit to practice.

We know that nine sutras done twice each with a 15-second interval will be about five minutes of samyama practice. If our session is coming in around five minutes, we will be on track. If it is significantly shorter or longer, we can make an adjustment. Over a few days or weeks the approximate 15-second interval can be achieved in that way.

For extended use of our last sutra for five minutes (*Akasha – Lightness of Air,* for most of us), we can go back to the same method of timing we use for deep meditation, rather than counting repetitions. So we just go on with the sutra with the approximate 15-second intervals until five minutes have passed. Having established the 15-second interval with our other sutras, we can be reasonably confident that we will remain on track with our last sutra for the five minutes at the end of the session.

From our own experience, we will find that 15 seconds is about the right amount of time for a sutra to be released in inner silence, and enlivened from within to produce its given effect via the process of moving stillness. Then another repetition of the same or next sutra will be necessary to continue the process of cultivating moving stillness. The human mind and nervous system are pre-wired for this approximate duration of processing in samyama, much as they are pre-wired for about 20 minutes of deep meditation per session for most people.

If we go significantly shorter than 15 seconds between sutra repetitions, there will not be enough time for stillness to fully absorb and move from within the sutra. This is a common occurrence in samyama practice – going through the sutras without adequate time of letting go in-between repetitions. This happens when the mind is fully engaged, which we are all prone to have happening in our busy lives. But this is samyama, where letting go is essential. The thing to do is develop the habit of letting go and allowing inner silence do its work, not minding thoughts or other experiences that may come up. In time, we learn to trust the process. It works!

Think of it this way – each repetition is a fraction of a second of faintly picking up the sutra, and 15 seconds of letting go. So, what is samyama primarily about? Is it primarily about the sutras? No, it is about letting go!

The reason we do not deliberately go much beyond 15 seconds between repetitions is because our awareness is naturally coming back out into thoughts by then, and is looking for something to latch on to. Either that, or the mind will be wandering aimlessly after about 15 seconds. It is the nature of the mind. So we give it another sutra repetition at that point, and let go. Because samyama is an enjoyable process, the mind will be happy to go with the sutra into stillness again.

Sometimes we will lose track of the time and go way over 15 seconds. It can happen. That is covered next.

Is getting lost during samyama practice okay? And once I realize it has happened, what do I do?

Losing track of our sutras is common, even for advanced practitioners, due to ongoing purification and opening occurring in the nervous system. It can happen to anyone at any time, and there is nothing to worry about. When we realize we have wandered off from our sutra practice, we just easily come back to it, wherever we left off.

If we find ourselves in a blizzard of thoughts, we do not hang on to them or try to force them out. We just easily come back to our samyama practice whenever we realize we have wandered off into a stream of thoughts, or any other experience.

Of course, wandering off and coming back to our sutras after some time has passed can mean our overall time will be longer. That is fine if we have the time. If we run out of time, then we can end our session as necessary wherever we happen to be in the sutra sequence and lay down to rest. There will always be other sessions, so we do not have to fret about an interrupted sequence of sutras. It has been for a good cause – our purification and opening, and for the ongoing process of our enlightenment. Everyone goes through changing experiences in samyama. Over the long term, samyama practice tends to become more steady and stable, as inner purification and opening advance in our nervous system.

If we get lost during the five-minute session with our last sutra, we can just lie down and rest if our time is up, when we realize we have been off somewhere.

It is common for such variations to occur, and we don't have to be concerned. It is our long term practice that will make the difference, so any variations that occur we just take in stride and keep on with our twice-daily practice.

I have heard that concentration is one of the key elements in samyama, but you do not mention it. Why?

In the style of samyama we are doing here, we pick up the object, the sutra, with attention and let it go. That picking up is called *dharana*, the sixth limb of yoga. The letting go is *dhyana*, which is the dissolving of the sutra, the meditation component, the seventh limb of yoga. Absorbing of the released sutra into our inner silence is the *samadhi* element, the eighth limb.

It is important to recognize that when we are picking up the sutra in a very faint and fuzzy way, then all three limbs of yoga will be *coexisting at the same time*. This becomes very natural and easy as our inner silence becomes steady and stable from our well established deep meditation practice and increasing experience in samyama. So, samyama is all three aspects together, and this is the essential cause that yields the remarkable effects of samyama.

While it might seem ironic, the *clunky stage* we may experience for a few days or weeks when getting started in samyama practice is caused by too much fixation of the mind on the surface level of the sutra. In other words, too much *concentration*. Success in samyama comes from touching the sutra faintly with awareness and letting it go. It is that simple.

The word *dharana*, is often translated to mean *concentration*, and this is a reflection of how some traditions practice both meditation and samyama, at least at certain stages, riveting the mind on an object (like a mantra or sutra) until it wears out and falls into stillness. Hence the word *concentration*. But this is not how deep meditation and samyama are practiced in the AYP approach, so we do not use the word *concentration* in relation to practice to avoid confusion with techniques taught elsewhere. But we do talk about *concentration* in another way.

Concentration means *intense or complete attention*. As we advance in our practices and experiences, inner silence continues to rise and stabilize in us, with many benefits. One of those benefits is the ability to increasingly focus attention like a laser beam on any task or object for an extended period of time. In other words, over time, yoga vastly increases our power of concentration. This ability to concentrate is an *effect* of yoga practices, which, in turn, becomes a *cause* in all that we undertake in life. An increased ability to concentrate is a practical benefit coming from yoga – one of many.

Like so many things in spiritual life, the rise of concentration from undifferentiated inner silence is a seeming paradox. Yet it happens. The more awareness (inner silence) we have available within ourselves, the more we are able to focus our attention intensely on external tasks for long periods of time.

When we engage in the efficient process of samyama on a daily basis, the flow of inner silence outward takes on a much more active role in our life. In time, it becomes a vast outpouring of attention, positive energy, intelligence and love that can lead to remarkable achievements. It is the stuff of miracles!

I have been doing Buddhist meditation for years. Can I use this style of samyama with it?
The fuel of samyama is inner silence. Any meditation technique that cultivates inner silence will

be a support for samyama practice. So, Buddhist meditation will work to the extent that it cultivates inner silence. Typically, the best time for structured samyama practice is right after meditation, which is the time when the most inner silence is likely to be present. We always rest for 5-10 minutes after samyama practice (lying down is good) to facilitate the winding down of inner energy flow and purification in the nervous system that may be occurring deep inside. If we get up too quickly, there can be some irritability in daily activity.

Samyama also works outside sitting practices, and we will get into that in the next chapter. Suffice to say that our genius resides in stillness within us, and to the extent we are able to entertain our desires in stillness, the likelihood of their fulfillment will be greatly enhanced. Einstein, Newton, Mozart and many others stand as testaments to this fact. Where there is inner silence and the principle of samyama operating, there is genius. It is in all of us.

Is doing samyama for gaining personal power wrong? Is it dangerous?

Of all the ways we can seek to increase our power in the world, samyama is the least dangerous. This is because true samyama is not *projection*. It is not acquiring anything, or manipulating anything in the world. Samyama is *surrender* to the divine within us. There is no harm that can come from this, even if we are doing it for selfish reasons.

What is not done for selfish reasons anyway? Everything we do is for our own self, even if we are making great sacrifices for others. It is merely a matter of what we regard our self to be. When we become filled with the joy of pure bliss consciousness, we begin to find our own self in everything and everyone around us, and act accordingly. This is the direct result of daily practice of deep meditation and samyama.

So, if we have some egotistical desire for enlightenment, or for some powers to exercise in the world, this is fine. Learn deep meditation. Learn samyama, and go for it. What will happen as we continue with practices and act in the world is, we will expand from the inside. As we do, our view will expand, as will our sense of self and the quality of our actions. Then we will be projecting our personal desires less on others, and surrendering them more into stillness. What comes out from that will be divine flow, no matter what sort of impure thoughts we have been letting go inside. It is a natural process of purification. It is very simple. Samyama is *divine judo* that takes all desires and elevates them to divine status, which then manifest as all love and support for everyone around us. This kind of surrender is not weakness. It is the greatest strength that can be found in life, nourished by the infinite residing within us.

So the fear about samyama being abused and used for wrong purposes is a myth. It is not possible with right practice. We can say that samyama is *morally self-regulating*, meaning that the deeper we go into it, the more moral strength we will have coming out from within us. If it is not right practice, not letting go into stillness, it is not samyama, and the power coming out will be much less.

Samyama is not projection of personal power. If there is projection involved in a practice, it is something else. It can be misguided ego, the dark arts, whatever we want to call it. It isn't samyama. If there is a danger, it is in the personal projection of power. Many of the world's ills have come from this. Samyama is the great undoer of egocentric adventures that have caused so much misery in the world. Correct practice of samyama is infallible in its results. And incorrect practice of samyama will not work. It is very safe.

So, let's begin samyama, and all that our heart craves deep within will be given to us, and much more.

I am experiencing fast breathing and physical movements sometimes during samyama. What is it?

When we systematically let go of our sutras in samyama practice, inner silence will begin to move inside us in particular ways that reflect the flavor of the sutras we are using, giving rise to a variety of sensations, thoughts and feelings. These will be the result of *purification* occurring in our nervous system. The movement of inner silence outward can also be experienced as *energy* moving through us, which can give rise to physical symptoms, such as alterations in breathing and physical movements.

Sometimes we call physical symptoms *automatic yoga*, since they may resemble yogic maneuvers and breathing practices. By automatic yoga, we do not mean practices we must follow when they happen. The way we handle such symptoms is to neither favor them, nor try and push them out. We just easily favor the practice we are doing over such experiences. In this case, the easy procedure of our samyama practice.

It is possible for the symptoms to become dramatic, such as the body beginning to shake and hop on our meditation seat during the lightness sutra. If this happens, we should take necessary precautions to protect ourselves and the furniture, by avoiding such activity on a fragile bed and having suitable padding underneath ourselves on a solid surface during our samyama. While our practice might seem chaotic sometimes, there is a method to it, and a lot of intelligence manifesting from within along with the energy. Still, it is up to us to take whatever precautions we feel are necessary to assure our safety. This is true for all yoga practices, and is an aspect of *self-pacing*.

Physical movements are caused by the friction of inner energies moving through our not yet fully purified nervous system. The further along the path we go, the more purification and opening we will have, and the less likely extreme physical movements will be. Then the experiences will be more along the lines of abiding inner silence, ecstatic bliss and outpouring divine love.

Along the path of purification and opening, we can have all sorts of things going on. It goes with the territory, and we deal with things as they come up in ways that assure our ongoing progress with comfort and safety.

I am filled with bright light and pleasurable energy during samyama, and for some time after. Is this the right result?

This is another way our purification and opening can be experienced. It means we are experiencing inner energy flow with less friction involved, which can give rise to experiences of inner light and ecstasy. Such experiences can come and go along the path of inner purification and opening.

Having this kind of experience does not mean we have arrived. More than likely we will continue to have many ups and downs along the way. It is a preview of what our life will be like permanently in the long term. The main thing is to continue with daily practices, and favor that over any lovely experiences that might distract us from doing the very practices that have created the experiences.

There are good things happening. It is our practice that is causing these experiences, so always favor the practice.

Why do I feel edgy and irritable after my samyama practice sometimes?

Irritability can result if we are overdoing in our practices, or coming out too fast, not taking adequate rest at the end of our sittings. One of the most common causes of irritability in activity is getting up too soon after practices. So be sure to address that first. It is very important to take at least 5-10 minutes of rest after our samyama practice. If we have a place to lie down during this time, it is good.

If irritability persists after practices, even when we are taking good rest before getting up, it can be overdoing in our practices. In the case of samyama, if two repetitions of our sutras is leaving us with irritability, then we can drop back to one repetition for a few sessions and see if that will help. Or, if we have forged ahead and are doing more than two repetitions of our sutras, and are having difficulties in our daily activity, then we should scale back a bit until things stabilize.

Irritability can also be caused by overdoing in any of our practices, so it is good to take a broad view of all the practices we are doing, and consider making adjustments in the practices that are most likely causing the excess energy flow and purification.

We will discuss the art of *self-pacing* in our practices more in the next sections.

What is the ultimate purpose of doing samyama?

As mentioned, whatever our purpose may be, be it for self or others, it will be a good enough reason to begin samyama, assuming we have been cultivating a foundation of inner silence beforehand. From there, the process of samyama itself will take us steadily toward our own higher purpose. If we are looking for powers, samyama will deliver them, but not necessarily in the way we may be expecting. When we engage in samyama, we may not always get exactly what we want, but we will always get what we need to advance on our spiritual path.

Ultimately, samyama, in conjunction with our other yoga practices, will lead us to enlightenment, which is abiding inner silence, ecstatic bliss and outpouring divine love.

Symptoms of Purification and Opening

All spiritual progress is based on the natural processes of purification and opening within us that are stimulated by spiritual practices. The more effective our practices are, the more purification and opening will be occurring, and the more spiritual progress we will experience in all avenues of our life.

Once we have our routine of samyama going, the symptoms of progress can vary widely, depending on several factors:

- The degree of abiding inner silence we have.

- The effectiveness (simplicity) and regularity of our samyama practice.

- The unique matrix of obstructions we each have embedded in our nervous system, which is gradually being unwound as we travel along our spiritual path.

- The intensity of our desire to progress spiritually. We call this *bhakti* – which means devotion to our highest chosen ideal.

Actually, bhakti comes first, because it is desire that fuels all of our endeavors along our spiritual path. Without desire, not much will happen. It is desire that determines what we will be practicing and when, and, to a degree, the effectiveness of our practices. When our heart is calling for the divine, the divine responds in kind. This is well known throughout the world.

But we need not be dependent on bhakti alone. Only a little desire (even skeptical curiosity) that inspires us to engage in practices like deep meditation, spinal breathing pranayama and samyama will have far-reaching consequences in our progress. Spiritual practices greatly leverage our bhakti and bhakti greatly leverages our spiritual practices. The whole is much greater than the sum of the parts.

In the case of samyama, the stimulation is initiated at the most subtle level of our being, within pure bliss consciousness, our inner silence. In order for samyama to be successfully undertaken, inner silence must already be present. This is why we say that a regular routine of deep meditation is the primary prerequisite for samyama.

Symptoms

The symptoms of spiritual progress vary widely from person to person, and even within the same person over time, as purification and opening proceed along their natural course. As we evolve, so too do our experiences.

Experiences can be divided into two classes – those associated with the rise of inner silence, and those associated with the rise of ecstatic energy throughout the body. Deep meditation and samyama mainly stimulate the rise of inner silence. Spinal breathing pranayama, other forms of pranayama, tantric sexual practices, asanas, mudras and bandhas mainly stimulate ecstatic energy (also known as *ecstatic conductivity* or *kundalini*). The symptoms of progress we may experience generally follow these two lines – stillness and ecstatic energy – with a remarkable merging occurring as these two aspects of experience advance within us over time. Samyama plays a key role in this merging, as do our ongoing activities in daily life.

So, as we begin and carry on with our spiritual practices over time, what might we expect? The best attitude to have is to not expect much. Easier said than done. Yet, the less expectation we harbor about our practices and experiences the better we will fare in the long run. The less we are concerned about experiences and the more we favor the procedures of our practices the smoother things will go.

It is possible that we will have little going on in the way of experiences for a long time. This does not indicate a lack of progress. In fact, it could indicate few apparent obstructions in our nervous system. On the other hand, we could have a lot of dramatic symptoms with energy moving, body shaking, etc., and it could mean little in the ultimate sense – only that we have a lot of obstructions dissolving in our nervous system.

So which is better? Neither. Every journey is unique, and equally valid. If we just keep going, favoring our practices over whatever may or may not be happening, we each will continue to progress at a good rate on our journey of purification and opening.

Having said that, let's look at some typical experiences. These will be a blend of the rise of stillness and ecstatic energy, which is often the case – experiences are often a mixed bag. As a general rule, any time we begin a new practice, we will go through a *clunky stage*, which will gradually settle down and stabilize as our nervous system acclimates to the purification and opening. Depending on how that process is proceeding, we may experience any or all of the following symptoms (or increases in them) as a result of adding samyama to our over all routine of practices:

- Inner peace, equanimity, abiding stillness, a sense of watching or witnessing our mind, emotions and events in the outer world.

- Spontaneous ecstatic pleasure occurring in the body. It may seem sexual, but not necessarily centered in the sexual organs.

- Inner non-physical sensory experiences involving sight, sound, touch, taste or smell. These experiences can also occur in relation to the physical environment, inside or outside the body, in the form of sweet tastes or smells, objects appearing luminous, finer values of sound (especially music), etc.

- A sense of oneness with the surroundings. More loving feelings in all relationships.

- A natural flow and effortlessness in activity. A sense of being supported from all sides. Events seeming beyond our control leading to positive outcomes.

- Feelings of energy moving in the body, sometimes pleasurable, sometimes not.

- Sudden physical movements, "automatic" yoga postures, rapid breathing or vibrations, lurching or hopping on the practice seat, etc.

- Temporary discomfort in the head, pelvic region or other areas of the body.

This is not an all-inclusive list, but covers the basic kinds of symptoms of purification and opening that can occur. None of these symptoms are prerequisites for progress on our path. The same purification can be occurring without any symptoms occurring at all. Everyone will be a bit different in how the path is traveled internally, so please temper expectations toward favoring practices over experiences, no matter what may be happening or not happening.

Experiences can be like *sirens*, and this is why we always easily favor the practice we are doing over any experiences that may come up, no matter how dramatic they may be.

<u>Experiences do not produce spiritual progress. Practices do.</u>

Because samyama is a process of cultivating our inner silence to move, the symptoms resulting from samyama practice can take on the characteristics of either inner silence or ecstatic energy moving, or both.

Samyama gives rise to a spiritual paradox – *moving stillness*. So, we may notice inner peace and equanimity after our samyama, even as we are feeling ecstatic energy movements. In fact, samyama can produce extremes of both aspects of experience at the same time. When added to abiding inner silence, samyama is a very powerful practice that reaches across the full spectrum of purification and opening within every cell of our body, and far beyond.

Self-Pacing

For centuries, many of the practices of yoga have been kept secret from all but a few. One of the reasons for this has been the assumption that most people are not capable of managing the process of purification and opening associated with spiritual practices such as samyama. It has been assumed that ordinary people are not able to stay focused enough to continue on the path in the face of the many experiences that can come up.

In the years since the AYP writings first came out, it has been found that, while this assumption may have been true in the past, it is not the case anymore. In fact, the opposite has been found to be true – the more knowledge practitioners have available on practices and the resulting experiences, the less likely they will be to have difficulties. Conversely, the less knowledge they have (fostered by secret teachings), the more prone they will be to overdo with incomplete practice routines and run into trouble.

A mainstay of the AYP approach to open source integrated spiritual practices is *self-pacing*.

Self-pacing is regulating our practices in a way that provides for good spiritual progress with comfort and safety. It is very simple.

If we are overly enthusiastic about our samyama and attempting to accelerate our progress with more repetitions of our sutras, we may find at some point that we are overdoing it – going beyond what our nervous system can assimilate in a given time period. The signal will be symptoms of excess – a headache, some irritability during the day, any of the previously listed symptoms taken to uncomfortable excess. Then we know it is time to back off on our practices a bit.

This does not mean stopping completely, except in extreme cases. More than likely, just backing off to a more modest routine of sutra repetitions will do the trick and bring things back into balance. As we get better at self-pacing, we will know to back off before things become excessively uncomfortable, just as we know to slow down when driving a car *before* we come to a sharp curve in the road.

In some cases where purification and opening are extreme, we may feel compelled to stop samyama for a few days or weeks. This is perfectly acceptable, as necessary. There is no point in struggling through with a full practice routine if we have gotten into an uncomfortable imbalance. We just regulate things to suit the situation, and allow our inner condition to normalize. There are other means we can apply to bring the inner energies into balance. These are covered elsewhere in the AYP writings where the management of *kundalini* is discussed. Sometimes it takes some special measures to cope with the purifying creative energies pouring out through us.

If we are prudent in self-pacing of our practices, extreme symptoms will be rare, and we will be able to move along at our own best pace. Everyone is different in how their process of purification and opening will unfold, so it is up to each of us to take responsibility for our practices and regulate them accordingly. We are conditioning our neurobiology for higher functioning, and we have our own unique journey to travel. This is what self-pacing is for – maximizing individual progress while maintaining good comfort and safety.

It should be mentioned that by the time we have added samyama to our practice routine, we will most likely be familiar with deep meditation, spinal breathing pranayama and other practices in the AYP integrated system. As part of this familiarity we will have developed a good practical knowledge of self-pacing as well, and be well familiar with using it in relation to our other practices.

Samyama is just another practice that we are adding into the mix, a practice that will accelerate our progress, taking us to a new level. In the case of self-pacing samyama, we can temporarily reduce the number of repetitions of our sutras until an energy excess has passed, and then step back up accordingly. If we get down to one repetition of our sutras, and it is still too much, then we can back off to one samyama session per day for a while. If this is still too much, we can discontinue samyama entirely for a few days or weeks. We can always come back when we have gotten past the rough spot in the road of purification and opening.

What we do not do is try and force our way through a period of excess purification and opening. While in the physical world of deeds, more concentrated effort can often lead to more progress, just the opposite is the case with spiritual practices. If we increase practices in the hope of blasting through to the other side of symptoms of excessive purification we are experiencing, it can set us back for a long time.

There is only so much purification the nervous system can tolerate in a given period of time. Our self-pacing has to be implemented around that reality. If we overdo persistently, we can become so uncomfortable that we can lose our motivation to practice altogether. That is the greatest risk in overdoing – falling off the path of practices completely due to the extreme discomfort that can result from pushing too hard in the face of excessive purification already occurring. Blasting through with practices does not work.

Let's drive smart and slow down when going into the sharp curves so we will not go flying off the cliff on the outside of the curve. Then we can speed up again as we come out of the curve and continue along on our journey with good progress and safety. If we understand self-pacing, we can make good progress no matter what sort of rough spots we may encounter along the way. It is common sense.

If we are doing samyama as part of a well developed routine including yoga postures (asanas), spinal breathing pranayama, deep meditation, mudras, bandhas, and other practices, self-pacing can be applied to any part of our routine, depending on which practice may be causing excess purification and opening. If we have been methodical in building up our practice routine over time, we will have a good familiarity with each of the practices we are using, and know how each one affects us. And as we add on, the combination of practices we are doing will have its own characteristics, which we are well familiar with, and be propelling us along our path at a rapid rate. This is why it is essential to build our practices up in a step-by-step fashion, allowing plenty of time for each practice to settle in before taking on a new one. If we do this, self-pacing will become a natural part of our path along the way, and we will have a good familiarity with the principles by the time we are engaging in samyama. We should not take on new practices before we are stable in our previous practices. This is an essential part of self-pacing also.

As we move forward on our path, we can continue to take advantage of the principle of self-pacing as we always have, applying it judiciously to whichever practice we may be overdoing at a given point in time. In some cases, there could be several practices we will be self-pacing at the same time.

All of the practices we are doing are interconnected through our nervous system, so we are obliged to take a holistic view of our yoga every step along the way. This is implemented by mastering the art of self-pacing. The more advanced we become, the more we will rely on our skills in self-pacing.

The more we understand yoga, the more we will understand ourselves and our path of purification and opening. That is because the human nervous system is the source of all yoga, and all spiritual progress. We are the doorway to the infinite.

Rise of the Active Witness

We have been discussing the characteristics of our spiritual unfoldment from two points of view – the rise of inner silence and the rise of ecstatic conductivity. While the symptoms of these two aspects of our nature are different, they ultimately lead to a merging.

There is a tendency in the various traditions to focus on either stillness or ecstatic energy, but not always on both and the merging of the two.

It is the reflection of a philosophical dichotomy that exists. One philosophical view is of a *non-dual* existence consisting of only one reality of stillness or emptiness, denying the reality or existence of the physical world. The other philosophical view is of a *dual* existence, where stillness or emptiness exists within the physical energetic universe of our everyday experience.

Whatever the truth of either of these philosophical points of view, we are fortunate to be able to experience reality within ourselves, and describe it from our own point of view. In other words, the truth will likely not be found in a philosophical description or point of view, but only by direct experience. Interestingly, both the *non-dual* and *dual* points of view can be affirmed by the same experience of human spiritual transformation!

Samyama is one of the great equalizers in this, because it begins in stillness, the non-dual, and *moves stillness* outward into our everyday actions, what we have previously known as the duality of life. When we see all *goodness* rising from within us in a unitary way, all debates about the true nature of life and existence evaporate. We can believe in our own experience.

This can also be called the rise of the *active witness*, meaning that quality in us which is the untouched and unmoving observer, becoming increasingly integrated in our everyday activities of the world. What has been known in the beginning as an unmoving static awareness, or inner witness, gradually becomes a dynamic ecstatic flow of positive qualities into our outer life. It is the direct experience of *Oneness* in diversity. How can this be? It is a mystery.

Well, it may be a mystery, but it is the key to enlightenment. It is also the resolution of the non-dual versus dual argument, for both will be right. Life becomes known as *One*, even as it continues in all of its variety before us. We can then see the non-dual nature of life, for all is but a play of the *One*. At the same time, we cannot deny the existence of that play, so the *One* is two also. Experientially, it is both non-dual and dual!

By cultivating *both* inner silence and ecstatic conductivity in our nervous system, and blending and moving them outward through the systematic practice of samyama, the truth of existence becomes known, and consciously lived in everything we do.

This is the rise of the active witness.

Chapter 3 – Expanded Applications

Our discussion of samyama so far has been focused on the practical application of its essential principles for broad purification and opening within our nervous system to advance our progress toward enlightenment. The incorporation of samyama into our daily routine of sitting practices right after deep meditation, and the selection of sutras to use, are designed to cover a wide territory both within and around us. We can say that this approach is *qualitative*, meaning it is for enhancing the quality of our life in the broadest terms. In doing so, it opens the door for improving our experience in everyday living – often in ways we might least expect. By steadily awakening the qualities of the divine within us, all of life is uplifted as we gradually become a channel for that expression.

With a good foundation of daily samyama practice in place, well stabilized within our overall routine of practices for some time, we will find ourselves in a position to consider further applications of samyama. Indeed, it is natural to desire more, building on the practice routine we have so prudently established. Fortunately we can do this in ways that do not overwhelm our schedule and busy life. We seek a good balance between our practices and daily living. We need both to assure our spiritual progress.

Here we will explore several expanded applications of samyama that can provide additional benefits in our daily life, without greatly increasing our time in practices each day. Indeed, much of what we will be adding here will be enhancing practices we are already doing, without adding any time to our twice-daily routine.

The applications of samyama we will discuss here are decidedly more *quantitative*, designed to enhance the flow of pure bliss consciousness on the physical plane in specific ways. None of these should be considered to be a replacement for our primary samyama practice as discussed in the previous chapter. Rather, these are logical expansions in practice that bring benefits in addition to our core sitting samyama practice.

Sooner or later we will find ourselves moving naturally into the areas discussed in this chapter. Perhaps we have been already. All of yoga will be percolating within us as we continue to advance along our path of daily practice.

Cosmic Samyama and Yoga Nidra

It has been said that the entire cosmos is contained within each of us. Perhaps that is what is meant by the phrase, "Humanity is created in God's image."

Regardless of what has been postulated by mystics, theologians and philosophers, it is a fact that most everyone at one time or other in this life has felt a kinship with the whole of creation. As we undertake deep meditation, spinal breathing pranayama, samyama and other yoga practices, this feeling of *Oneness* gradually increases, in time becoming a full time experience.

Somewhere along the way, we might ask, "Is there a way to accelerate this rising sense of unity I am feeling?"

If we continue our practices, it will most certainly continue to grow, for it is only ourselves we are discovering. Whatever *That* is, we will come to know it by direct experience. No one else's word has to be taken as gospel. Direct experience will tell the tale. So let's move on to that.

There is an additional procedure of samyama we can utilize that can enhance two aspects of our unfoldment.

First is aiding in the perception of our cosmic dimensions. This is applying samyama in a way that is *quantitative*, meaning we are addressing and integrating the furthest reaches of our physical dimensions in samyama practice.

Second is enhancing our experience of *yoga nidra*, which means *yogic sleep*. Yoga nidra is not primarily about sleep really. It is about further stabilizing our inner silence, the witness, which is known to coexist with our other states of consciousness – waking state, dreaming sleep state, and deep dreamless sleep state. When we are awake, we tend to call inner silence the *witness*, among other things. In sleep, inner silence is also called *yoga nidra*, or *yogic sleep*. It is the same thing.

Inner silence is also called *turiya*, which means the *fourth state*, which can be present during any of the other three states – waking, dreaming sleep or deep sleep. The further we go along the path of yoga, the more inner silence we will have present all the time, twenty-four hours per day, seven days per week (24/7).

The new procedure of samyama we are introducing here bears some resemblance to so-called *guided meditation* methods that are used to promote yoga nidra. So, some might say, "Oh, this is a yoga nidra practice. AYP is finally offering a yoga nidra practice!"

But, it isn't really, because this is not an externally guided meditation practice. It is self-directed and can be done anywhere without external assistance, recordings or other props. Only your nervous system is needed. It involves the systematic use of samyama, which is another major difference from the multitude of externally guided meditation practices out there.

We will call it *cosmic samyama.*

The Practice of Cosmic Samyama

Cosmic samyama expands our sense of physical presence within and beyond our body. This is an expansion of our awareness in a way that transcends the physical, while cultivating the yoga nidra effect. The more cosmic we become, the more we become *infinite awareness*, not bound by any physical dimensions. As we expand our awareness to encompass all that is physical, the physical evaporates into the vastness of our inner space. It is one of those paradoxes we find in yoga. The paradox is resolved by direct experience, so let's get into it.

First, it is recommended that cosmic samyama not be undertaken until our regular sitting samyama practice (Chapter 2) is well-established and stable for at least several months, preferably longer. Each new practice we add brings new layers of purification and opening in our nervous system. This is a good thing. But if we do not stabilize each practice before taking on the next one, there can be excessive energy flow, discomfort, and the necessity to discontinue some or all of our practices for a time. Obviously, this does not foster progress. So, the best course in taking on new practices is a measured one. Keep in mind that the full effects of inner purification and opening with any new practice will take months to be realized – sometimes years. So, please do step carefully and always remember to self-pace. The more advanced we become, the more important prudent self-pacing becomes.

Cosmic samyama is a practice we will do while lying on our back, relaxed with eyes closed. It is similar to the corpse pose utilized at the end of yoga asanas, except we elevate our head on a pillow or two and rest our hands easily on our solar plexus, the area between the navel and the bottom of the ribs. Our legs can lie flat and easy. This can be done on the bed, if desired. If we are not in a place where we are able to lie down, then we just lean back in whatever place we happen to be sitting. The key thing is to be comfortable.

Cosmic samyama can be performed at the end of our sitting practices, using a predetermined series of sutras. It then becomes the first part of our rest period after all of our sitting practices are finished. We also have the option to do it right before we go to sleep at night.

The practice is similar to our regular sitting samyama routine, with an additional element – the physical location of awareness with the sutras. We use a specific sequence of sutras for cosmic samyama and use them in the same way every time we practice. We go through them once, with one repetition of each sutra. When we pick up each sutra, we let our awareness naturally go to the location the sutra is associated with. When we let go of the sutra for the 15-second interval, we do it from the designated location of the sutra, allowing our attention to release from that location. The result will be an expansion of awareness from that location.

For example, the first sutra we use in cosmic samyama is *Feet*. When we lie down at the end of our sitting practices, we relax for a minute or two, and then pick up the first sutra, *Feet*. At the same time we pick up the location of our feet. As soon as we have picked up the sutra at the designated location, we let it go. As with sitting samyama, picking up the sutra (and location in this case) is faint and fuzzy. We let it go at the location of our awareness, at the feet. From there it is in the hands of our inner silence. We may feel some expansion occurring in the area of our feet. Or maybe not. Whatever happens will be taken care of by our inner silence. When about 15 seconds have passed, we go on to the next sutra, and so on all the way through, with one repetition of each sutra at the designated location, and letting go.

We have 16 sutras for cosmic samyama. When we have completed the series, in about five minutes or so, we rest for at least another five minutes to allow the effects of our samyama to stabilize before we get up. If we feel some irritability after we are out of practices for a while, it will be a possible sign of not taking enough rest before getting up.

Let's list all of the sutras now, along with indications of their corresponding locations, as applicable. For those whose first language is not English, these sutras may be translated as desired for easiest recognition.

- **Feet** – both feet

- **Knees** – both knees

- **Root** – perineum/anus

- **Sex** – center of pelvic region

- **Navel** – navel/solar plexus area

- **Heart** – center of chest behind the breastbone

- **Throat** – hollow of throat

- **Eye** – center brow, extending back to center of head and down into the brain stem

- **Crown** – a point one hand's width (five fingers) above the top of head

- **Earth**

- **Moon**

- **Sun**

- **Solar System**

- **Galaxy**

- **Cosmos**

- **Unbounded Awareness**

When using these sutras, we do not repeat the location description mentally, only the sutra itself. So when picking up the word *Feet*, we do not think "both feet." We just let our attention embrace both feet, and then let go of both sutra and physical location of attention from there. All of this very faint and fuzzy. Likewise, when we pick up the word *Knees*, we do not think "both knees." We pick up the sutra at the location of both knees and let go. And so on…

No doubt it is noticed that no location is given for the sutras from *Earth* onward. So where is *Earth*? Is it the Earth we are on, teeming with life, or is it the lovely blue ball seen from a distance in vast empty space both outside and inside us. It is all of these, so we don't specify a location. Earth is Earth, and we use the sutra only. The word contains all that Earth is, including its location. The same goes for *Moon*, *Sun*, *Solar System*, *Galaxy* and *Cosmos*. Where are all of these things? They are in us and around us in the vastness of infinite inner and outer space. So we use them as sutra words only. Deep in inner silence, we know them intimately.

And where is *Unbounded Awareness*? Well, it is the same as *Cosmos*, yes? Everywhere within us and around us. So we just pick up the outer space/inner space sutras for what they are, using our normal samyama technique, and we will have the result.

While it takes millions of years for light to traverse the physical universe, we can instantly encompass and manifest everything from within our pure bliss consciousness with the simple technique of cosmic samyama. Recall that cosmic samyama is for integrating our inner and outer physical dimensions in consciousness. Inner and outer are the same. Even though we are infinite both inside and outside, there is no distance or time. Our awareness contains all of space and time. On the level of our samyama practice, the *now* of pure bliss consciousness is everything, and everything pours out from *That*.

The expansion of awareness utilizing the cosmic samyama sutras is by orders of magnitude to the infinite, both within us and outside us. Our wondrous Earth is but a speck in our solar system. Our sun is one of billions in our galaxy. And our galaxy is infinitesimally small in the vast cosmos. Yet, it is all contained within us – within our unbounded awareness. The cosmos is us, and we are the cosmos.

In engaging in cosmic samyama, we are dissolving the yogic paradox – the entire cosmos and all of eternity consciously contained within this human form, this human being, this consciousness of ours. Cosmic samyama is for advancing our direct experience of *That*.

A noticeable effect of this inner and outer cosmic merging is the stabilization of unbounded awareness. So much so that we may find ourselves becoming absorbed in it. This is normal. It is the quality of yoga nidra. Once we complete our rest period and get up from our cosmic samyama, the deep silence and sense of cosmic universality we have gained will be carried out into our daily activity, and influence our actions accordingly. Cosmic samyama and yoga nidra are not a departure from this world. Rather, through cosmic samyama and yoga nidra, the infinite is brought into this world through us, and into our every action.

If we find ourselves wandering off during cosmic samyama practice, we just easily pick up where we left off. If we do wander off, it can be into a state of unbounded awareness. We might feel that we are asleep, but fully awake inside at the same time. This is *yoga nidra – yogic sleep*. It is a common experience in cosmic samyama. We are, after all, the infinite pure bliss consciousness behind it all. If we have wandered off and time has run out by the time we realize we have not completed our sutras, it is okay to discontinue our sutras, take some rest and get up. Or, if we have time, we can continue to the end of our sutras, no matter how long it takes.

It is also common to become absorbed in yoga nidra for some time during rest after our cosmic samyama practice. If we drift off into yoga nidra after our morning or afternoon practice, we will get up feeling extra refreshed. If we have practiced at bedtime, this is a great way to go to sleep. We may be watching ourselves restfully sleeping all night. It's a good thing. However, cosmic samyama is not recommended to be used in combination with so-called *lucid dreaming* practices. This can cause imbalances in the nervous system leading to sleep deprivation, which is not beneficial for our health and wellbeing. If sleep deprivation is occurring in relation to cosmic samyama, then self-pacing of the practice should be applied. We need our sleep!

Cosmic samyama gradually cultivates an enhanced foundation of inner silence during our daily activities, and a much greater sense of unity in all that we undertake. This is a big boost to all of our other yoga practices as well, including our sitting samyama practice.

If we experience excess energy flow occurring as a result of our cosmic samyama, we self-pace accordingly, like we do with any of our practices. Because we are using one repetition for each sutra and location, self-pacing of cosmic samyama would mean reducing the number of sessions in a day. So, if we are doing cosmic samyama after both of our sitting practice routines, and again at bedtime, and are having too much purification occurring during the day (usually in the form of irritability) or at night (as sleeplessness), then we can reduce the number of sessions for a while until there is stabilization.

We may find that cosmic samyama, itself, offers additional balance, reducing energy imbalances within the body related to overdoing in other yoga practices. Cosmic samyama expands and balances the flow of our energies between inner and outer expression, reducing the congestion that can occur within the nervous system. This balancing effect is delicate, and depends largely on the degree of purification having been previously achieved at the crown with our other practices. This is why it is preferable to have a stable routine of sitting practices well established prior to undertaking cosmic samyama. From there, we can proceed with our expanded opening, reaching far within and beyond the physical body. Then we may find that cosmic samyama serves as a stabilizing factor for everything else that is going on inside us.

The sutras we are using in cosmic samyama are universal points of awareness that unfold our infinite dimensions, inside and outside our body. As we move ahead, we will find both to be aspects of the same reality, all manifesting from the same infinite sea of our unbounded silent awareness, like waves on the great ocean. We are that ocean.

Samyama and Yoga Postures (Asanas)

For those who are established in doing a daily routine of yoga postures (asanas), samyama can be incorporated in a way that can enhance the effects of our bending and stretching.

In the AYP approach, a concise sequence of yoga postures is used before our twice-daily sessions of sitting practices. We will use this routine as a baseline for incorporating samyama into yoga postures. Samyama can be incorporated into any other routine of yoga postures in a similar fashion.

For those who are well established in their sitting samyama practice after deep meditation, it is easy to add samyama to asanas. Our habit of touching a word or phrase (sutra) faintly with attention and letting it go into stillness will gradually show up in many avenues of our life, with great benefit. So it can be in our structured asana routine as well.

If we take the approach of initiating a descriptive name, or sutra, for each asana as we are first entering the posture, and let go of the sutra while we are in the posture, this is all that is necessary.

Having let go of the sutra, our attention will naturally go with the posture and expand beyond it, adding a far greater component of inner silence to the posture than was there before adding samyama. The result of this is more relaxation during the posture, more lasting effects, and a smoother performance of the physical posture itself. Keep in mind that we never force in yoga postures, always going to our comfortable limit, and not beyond into discomfort. This is the primary instruction in all yoga practices – never force.

In the AYP approach, the duration of most of our postures is in the 10-15 second range, and this is a good fit with the release of sutras into our inner silence. In the case of samyama during yoga postures, we are engaging *stillness in action*, literally. As we continue to develop this kind of habit in our thinking and doing, it will have profound implications in our daily life. There is great power in it.

Here are the names of the yoga postures we use in the AYP approach, which can be used as sutras for the corresponding postures. These can be translated to suit language. The Sanskrit names can also be used, if the meanings are clear to us in terms of the physical attributes of the postures.

For instructions on yoga postures, see *Asanas, Mudras and Bandhas – Awakening Ecstatic Kundalini*, or the *AYP Easy Lessons* book.

 Warm-up, head to heart

 Warm-up, arms to heart

 Warm-up, legs to heart

 Knees to chest roll

 Kneeling seat

Sitting, head to left knee
(then – Sitting, head to right knee)

 Sitting, head to both knees

 Shoulder stand

 Plow

 Seal of yoga

 Cobra

 Locust

 Spinal twist left
(then – Spinal twist right)

 Abdominal lift

 Standing back stretch

 Standing toe touch

 Corpse

These sutras can be adjusted as needed if and when our asana routine is modified, as would be the case when using the AYP abbreviated asana routine (covered in the above referenced books), or as we may add more advanced postures over time. All we need is a word or short phrase that cues our inner silence to the performance of the posture. Remember, a sutra is a code that we easily release into stillness. Inner silence will do the rest.

What we may find with the use of samyama in yoga postures is that our comfortable limit moves, giving us a bit more reach than we may have expected. This is good, but do not take it as a signal to push beyond whatever that expanding comfortable limit may be. Even with the advantage of samyama, we are obliged to prudently observe the principles of self-pacing in every aspect of our yoga practices.

The addition of samyama to our asana routine can greatly enhance the effects of our postures physically, emotionally and mentally. When using asanas as a warm-up for our sitting practices, adding samyama enhances the relaxation of our nervous system, setting us up for deeper practice of spinal breathing pranayama, deep meditation, sitting samyama, and our other practices.

Prayer and the Principles of Samyama

Prayer is the most commonly used spiritual practice in all of the religious traditions around the world. Prayer comes wrapped in many forms of culture and ritual. Yet, it is essentially the same practice everywhere. It involves placing attention on an object, or series of objects, repetition, and surrender of the object(s) to the divine.

Does this sound familiar? It should. It is the application of the principles of samyama. It should not be a surprise. The principles of samyama are universal and are contained within all of us. They are found manifesting in prayer practice in every religious tradition. The principles of samyama are inherent in everyone, and for this reason prayer has been found to work, more or less, for thousands of years.

What do we mean by, "Prayer works, more or less"?

Certainly, all prayers are not answered to our satisfaction. The more we are externally invested in the particular outcome desired from prayer, the less likely that specific outcome will be forthcoming. This is because the cultivation of expectations for a specific outcome is not true prayer (or samyama). Expectations are external projections of the mind that have little to do with prayer. Our personal desires will short-circuit the divine outflow.

On the other hand, it will be a different story if we offer a specific object in our prayers and release it to inner silence (the divine) within us without hanging on to expectations. This will always lead to a result, not necessarily exactly what we expected, but something fruitful all the same. What comes from prayer is a function of our surrender, not our expectation. This is the key point in all prayer.

<u>Surrender of the object to the divine is the essential operating principle in prayer</u>.

This is beautifully expressed in the Biblical phrase, "Thy will be done."

This is not an invitation to lead a passive life without active participation. Real surrender is not passive. It is tremendously dynamic. It is the rise of the active witness. It is the birth of stillness in action. All sorts of miraculous events will flow out of this kind of awakening – this kind of active surrender.

Effective prayer is effective *relationship* with the divine within us. It is dynamic relationship. In this kind of relationship, the attention is brought to many objects, sometimes in structured practice and sometimes spontaneously. With the rise of stillness in action, the natural flow of desires is steadily elevated, and so are the objects selected, which are released into stillness. And the divine flow pours out from within, increasing from its own momentum, like a snowball rolling downhill. Active surrender!

Our own activity in daily living is part of this process. We can be very active, pursuing our goals in life, and in surrender at the same time. As a matter of fact, the more active we are in moving toward our goals, the more effective our spiritual practices and prayers will be. There is the expression, "The Lord helps those who help themselves." It is true. This is especially applicable for those who are engaged in daily spiritual practices, because stillness becomes very active, and this means action in the form of outpouring divine energy.

When we speak of the *object* of our prayer, we can apply some additional useful knowledge from the principles of samyama by considering the application of the concept of *sutra*. Recall that a sutra is a *code word* or *phrase* that contains meaning stored deep in our consciousness in the seeds of our language. If we have understood a sutra before we enter samyama practice, we will not have to be understanding it during samyama practice. We just pick it up and let it go. The word or phrase will contain the meaning. This is a highly effective way to release content into stillness, including in prayer. We are shrinking the proverbial camel, so it can pass easily through the eye of the needle into stillness. From there, inner silence will take over.

Practical Prayer with Samyama

Let's consider a practical example. If we have a dear relative or friend who is ill, we may wish to offer a prayer for them. We know their name, and that they are ill. Deep within us we have the essence of who they are. It is contained deep in our consciousness.

So, what is the best way to offer a prayer for this person? Does it have to be a long, drawn out prayer? If so, how would we surrender such a long and drawn out petition into stillness? While our prayer may be rich in words, how can we cram all of that richness through the eye of the needle into stillness? Stillness does not need our elaborate words. More is less in this case.

It is much better to do a simple repetition of the person's name, faintly picking it up and releasing it into stillness, letting it go for about 15 seconds, and then touching the name again on the boundary of stillness in a very faint way. Then we can let it go again. And again, for as many times as we feel appropriate, but not to the point of excess and strain. Everything we know about the person and all that is needed to enliven divine healing energy is contained in the simple procedure of releasing their name into divine stillness. We can be certain that divine healing energy will be stirred by our prayer. It is very simple.

5-10 minutes is a good period to engage in a prayer when applied with samyama. It will be very powerful, particularly if we have been cultivating inner silence through deep meditation beforehand. Therefore, a good time to engage in such prayer activity is soon after our sitting practices. If this is not the case, then 5-10 minutes of deep meditation right before prayer will help stabilize a good initial condition of inner silence. If we do this, our prayer will be more powerful.

The degree of help that may be received by another is also dependent on the degree of receptivity, so it is good for the person in need to be aware of the prayers being offered on their behalf. Receptivity is the greater half of the equation. If this were not so, sincere prayers would have much greater effect than is often the case. If the recipient is open and receptive, the entire universe will run to fill the need. As has been said, "Your faith has made you whole."

It will be a good idea to take some extra rest after doing samyama-style prayer. Keep in mind that while we are helping others, we are also advancing our own inner purification and opening, so some rest afterward is advised to avoid the possibility of some irritability occurring when we get up and go out into our daily activities.

The same kind of procedure can be used with traditional prayers, meditating first for 5-10 minutes, and then picking up each phrase or line of our traditional prayer faintly and releasing it into stillness, letting go for about 15 seconds before picking up the next phrase or line. It can be done while using a rosary or mala also.

In many traditions, group prayer is used to multiply the effects of individual prayer. When refining our prayer using the principles of samyama, and doing it in a group, the effects can be greatly amplified. It is not mandatory for a prayer group to be physically located in one place. It has been found that a coordinated prayer offered by many people in many locations, synchronized in time, is very powerful in its positive effects. With the advent of the Internet and instant worldwide communications, there are many possibilities for groups to work together in this way for the betterment of family, friends, and all of humanity.

Prayer with Samyama to Dissolve Global Problems
There are innumerable noble efforts going on around the world to relieve the suffering of humanity, and to prevent it in the future. So much of suffering is spawned from negative attitudes and thinking, which lead to harmful actions. Indeed, human beings in their present state seem to be obsessed with negativity.

Read or watch any summary of the daily news, and it will be overflowing with the three *D's* – disaster, death and despair. Is this the world we want? Nearly everyone agrees that we do not, and many are working directly to relieve the serious problems that the world faces.

And many are offering their prayers. When it comes to prayer, there is a way to greatly strengthen our influence over the problems of the world. Or, to be more specific, greatly increase the divine influence that comes from within all of us. We have the ability to dissolve the world's problems simply by giving our attention to them in an effective way, using the principles of samyama. From there, we may also be inspired to engage in further positive action in the world. Whether we are spurred to action or not, our influence will be felt simply by the fact that we have been praying in a way that is extremely powerful. Anyone can make a huge contribution to dissolving the world's problems in this way.

We have discussed previously how prayers can be greatly strengthened by condensing the content into sutras, which are code words that can be used in the systematic way described. This is how we release the full content of our prayer easily into our inner silence, where the infinite power of all *goodness* will manifest them back out in a positive way. This goes for any sutra we wish to devise. Whatever we surrender to our inner silence will come out with radiant power and purpose. In time, we come to know that we can count on this principle. As our experience and belief grow, so does the purifying power flowing from within us.

In the *Samyama Sutras of Patanjali* (see Appendix), the principle of surrendering obstructions to inner silence is presented, where we can do samyama directly on an obstruction (a negative influence) in order to remove it. Several examples can be found in the list of sutras in the Appendix. This supports the assertion that all sutras, regardless of content, will bring a positive effect when utilized within samyama.

In using a sutra that represents an obstruction (or group of obstructions) we do not have to specify what we want done with the obstruction. Inner silence knows what to do with the obstruction – dissolve it!

We can divide sutras into two categories:

Qualities – Sutras that manifest the enhancement of a designated quality, such as *Love* (from our core sutras – Chapter 2).

Obstructions – Sutras that, when released in inner silence, will dissolve the implicit obstruction, such as the sutra, *Unseen Obstructions* (from the Appendix).

In the AYP sutra lists we are using so far, the sutras represent qualities, for the most part. For dissolving the problems of the world, it can be effective to use sutras representing the obstructions to be dissolved, as these will be more specific in terms of what is to be acted upon by pure bliss consciousness.

A few that will be familiar include *Ignorance, Poverty, Hunger, Disease, Fear, Hatred, War...*

We can make each of these painfully more specific with a word or two added. Most will not need help with this. Just check the daily headlines. The bad news on obstructions can be good for something useful – samyama! We may feel the pain in just reading these words, which encapsulate so much suffering in the world. In samyama we will be more deeply moved as global impurities in the family of humanity are dissolving in pure bliss consciousness.

Tears may come to our eyes. It is our compassion coming up from deep inside. But we are not here to wallow in sentimentality, no matter how divinely inspired and well intentioned. We want to go much further. We want to dissolve these obstacles to global human enlightenment. And we can.

We can pray utilizing samyama on any or all obstructions to human happiness and global enlightenment, using the same method described previously. Meditate for 5-10 minutes, and then faintly touch the sutra and let it go into inner silence for about 15 seconds. And again, and again, continuing for 5-10 minutes. If we decide to use a series of sutras of our own choosing in this way, then we can repeat each sutra two, three or four times, depending on how many we are using and how long we want our session to last.

The effectiveness of our prayer will depend on following the procedure of samyama and on the consistency of our practice over days, weeks, months and years. The more consistent our practice, the more results we will produce.

As with prayers offered for individuals, the strength of prayers using samyama for dissolving global problems can be amplified by engaging in them at the same time in groups. This can be done with groups physically located in the same place or with groups widely dispersed geographically, using communications and coordination via the Internet.

However, do not feel that a group is mandatory to make a difference in dissolving the problems of the world. Groups help, but we can pray alone too. One persistent individual engaged in systematic samyama practice on a daily basis for weeks, months and years can move mountains, and transform world consciousness. So, if there is a desire to illuminate the world from within, there is no need to wait for a group to form. We can each start where we are – right here, right now. Indeed, thousands of people engaged in individual daily samyama practice constitute an ongoing group, whether everyone is practicing at the same time, or not. So, in truth, we will never be alone in our endeavors.

Just a reminder that it will be best to be well established in our sitting samyama routine before we engage in the application of samyama with prayers. It is very important to have a stable daily practice forming a good foundation, and to be methodical in implementing any samyama-related additions or modifications to any practice, including our daily prayers. Spiritual practices work best when they are scheduled (repeated daily) and systematic. Then we will have a good handle on what is happening in any given session, and can self-pace our practice accordingly.

As was mentioned at the beginning of this section, prayer is spiritual practice. With the principles of samyama added, the power of our prayers will be greatly intensified, producing purification and opening within us as energy moves in relation to that which we are praying for. We will know if we are overdoing by how we feel during and after practice. If there is irritability, we may need to add a rest period at the end of our prayer session, or self-pace (temporarily scale back) the practice as we would for any other spiritual practice we are doing that may be causing excess energy flow. While energy symptoms are a confirmation that we are making strides, we'd like to pace our progress to be comfortable and safe, to avoid having to back off practices completely for an extended period during a major overload. In this way, we can continue on an ongoing basis, dissolving obstructions to enlightenment within ourselves and within everyone around the world.

It is not necessary for anyone to alter their religious beliefs or customs to make good use of the natural principles of samyama that exist in all of us. Whatever our religion may be, our practice of prayer can be greatly enriched. By applying the simple and universal principles of samyama, our prayers can be empowered in ways that fulfill their purpose – maximizing the divine presence and influence in our life, and in the lives of people everywhere.

Samyama in Daily Living

The reason we do daily yoga practices is to improve the quality of our life outside practices. Otherwise, what would be the point? Certainly we are in it for more than the flashy experiences that may come and go while we are sitting in practices. These are merely the expression of inner purification and opening while it is occurring. The real test of our practices is in how we feel during the rest of our day, between our practice sessions. It is in daily activity that we will know what we are accomplishing with our yoga.

Moving Stillness and Active Surrender

Since we began deep meditation, we likely noticed an inner calm creeping up in our life over time, a sort of inner stillness that somehow sets us apart from the ups and downs of life. Something in us is able to observe all that is going on without being affected. We have called it the *witness*. It has many other names. It is a condition that has great practical value, because it enables us to remain calm and more collected throughout the storms of daily life.

Yet, having the witness in daily life is still a condition of duality. It is our silent self inside here, with all the stuff of life happening out there. So, what happens?

Stillness begins to move outward.

Why?

As paradoxical as it may sound, it is the nature of inner stillness to move. Indeed, all that exists on this material plane is the product of stillness moving. Keep in mind that all we see is the manifestation of bits of energy whirling in vast empty space. So, it is not untypical that we will find stillness moving from within us also. We have been evolving toward that eventuality for a long time. With the methods of yoga, we are able to accelerate the process significantly.

Samyama is a means for directly stimulating stillness to move in particular ways. If we combine a range of these particular ways using appropriate lists of sutras, we will develop the ability to move stillness in all ways, because our nervous system will become purified and opened in all directions. Just as conditioning our body with a broad set of physical exercises will enable us to engage in a variety of athletic activities, so too will a balanced daily samyama practice prepare us to become a channel of pure bliss consciousness in the world in many ways.

When we do our structured samyama practice, we are cultivating the habit of thinking, feeling and doing on the level of stillness. In daily activity, this gradually results in our inner silence, the witness, becoming active. As this occurs, stillness moves increasingly into all of our actions.

From a practical point of view, this means more effectiveness in daily activity – more flexibility, more energy, more creativity, more intuition, more patience, and so on. Underlying it all will be more love and compassion. This is why we say that samyama cultivates *outpouring divine love*.

All of this comes up as inner habit cultivated in our daily samyama practice. It is a new way of functioning that can greatly enhance the quality of our life, while positively influencing everyone around us at the same time.

And what is this habit? It is the habit of surrendering our thoughts, desires and feelings within silence.

Can we predict exactly what will come out of this? No, we can't. We can only know that the result will be dynamic and for the common good. There is a mystery in this. For those who develop the habit of surrender, life becomes filled with small miracles, and, sometimes, big ones. When these things happen, it is not by personal will. It is by divine outflow that all miracles happen, including all that we are witnessing in this glorious creation.

This is a path of *active surrender*. It is not a passive process. Surrender is not a non-doing. It is doing and letting go. This is the essence of samyama, whether we are engaged in structured sitting practices or going about our business in the world. We continue to act in daily life according to the natural flow of our inspiration and desires, surrendering all the while. Once we have cultivated the habit, we don't have to think about it as technique, because it becomes part of our normal functioning in daily living.

Natural Self-Inquiry

At some point, we may notice that we have developed the ability to reinforce our habit of surrender during daily activity. With inner silence (the witness) increasingly present in our life, we find ourselves in a position to observe our thoughts and feelings like objects moving through inner space. When we notice projections of thought that are subconsciously pre-constructed in ways that are harmful to us or to others, we can easily ask ourselves if this is in our best interest. As soon as we ask, the wayward thought or feeling will dissolve under the spyglass of pure bliss consciousness. Old knee-jerk habits of thinking that are not beneficial can be dissolved in this way as our steadfastness in stillness grows. We find that we have much greater influence over thoughts and feelings that may have bound us to unproductive living patterns in the past. This practice of consciously dissolving unproductive thinking patterns is called *self-inquiry*.

Through the habit of active surrender cultivated in deep meditation and samyama, combined with our ability to operate consciously within the increasing transparency of our inner world, we find our thoughts and feelings becoming the vehicles of outward flowing pure bliss consciousness.

Intentional Divine Flow

At the same time, the dynamics of stillness in action include the expansion of ecstasy. In fact, stillness in action rides on rising ecstatic conductivity surging up from within us, and overflowing to illuminate everything in our surrounding environment. The full effects of samyama are found when inner silence and ecstatic conductivity are merging to become *One*. Then, when we engage in the world, it will be increasingly from the point of view of ecstatic bliss and the outpouring of love that comes with it. As we become increasingly permeated by silence and ecstatic bliss in all that we do, every thought, word and deed becomes an act of samyama, which is living fully while letting go. It is an *intentional divine flow* with which we have become merged.

Transformation of Karmic Influences

As we come to live consciously in the natural outpouring of divine love coming through us, there will be very little we do that will not be in harmony with our continuing evolution and the evolution of all who are around us. Even the iron fist of karma will lose its grip on us. Does karma go away? Does it dissolve and disappear? No. It is transformed. Or, to put it more accurately, the *influence of karma* is transformed. This is because we have been transformed.

Keep in mind that the manifestation of karma in our life does not occur in a fixed inalterable way. While there are influences we all must live with, the manifestation of those influences are a function of our spiritual condition. The more closed down (blocked) our inner condition is, the more susceptible we will be to the forces that enter our life. We will be like a leaf being carried on the wind. We all have known the feeling, yes?

On the other hand, as we undergo purification and opening as a result of our long term daily spiritual practices, we will gradually become much less a leaf in the wind of karmic influences, and more a channel of karmic influences for higher purpose.

If our karma has had us on a date with disaster at some point in time, our spiritual practices will gradually be transforming that eventuality into a date with good providence. This is the transformation of karmic influences. As we transform ourselves spiritually, our fortunes will change in every way. There is no outside force that can alter this fact, because the human nervous system is the doorway to the divine. Once the door is open, all expression of energy on this earth will be for *That*, including all karmic influences.

The natural attunement of the principles of samyama (functioning as stillness in action) in all aspects of our daily life engages us perpetually in conscious participation with the divine flow. It is a condition of permanent happiness.

Siddhis – Super-Normal Powers

The possibility of ordinary human beings exhibiting extraordinary powers has always drawn public attention. Stories, myths and legends, both ancient and modern, depicting miraculous performances by heroes and villains alike never fail to find an audience. Everyone loves a super hero. Deep down, we all dream of becoming super heroes ourselves. Why? Because, while we may not believe we are capable of leaping tall buildings, we do sense our infinite inner dimensions and the possibilities associated with that. We are all wired that way.

It is natural for human beings to look beyond the status quo, as miraculous as that status quo may be in and of itself. All of life is, after all, a marvelous miracle.

Our accomplishments in applying natural laws, through applied science for the betterment of humankind, stand as testament to our capabilities. Yet, what we know and have applied so far doesn't even scratch the surface of what is to come. There is more that we do not know than there is that we do know. Of this we can be certain. So, are human beings capable of super-normal powers? Well, why not? We won't know for sure until we investigate further. Much further. If we do so within the context of promoting the natural process of human spiritual transformation, we will not go too far wrong – powers or no powers.

It should not be a surprise that the religions and spiritual traditions of the world have always dangled siddhis, miracles and extraordinary experiences as carrots to attract followers to their fold. This is not a reflection on the possibility, or lack thereof, of super-normal powers. It is just good marketing.

Most of the scriptures of the world contain exhibitions of super-normal powers, usually with the proviso that such things *come from God*. Even so, as eager aspirants, we often will seek the acts themselves before attempting to join with the primal cause – the divine within us.

Patanjali, one of the greatest integrators of spiritual practices of all time, hangs out the carrot in one whole chapter (out of four) in his ancient and very famous *Yoga Sutras*. At the same time he tells us, "Don't get too attached to these things."

Nevertheless, we read his chapter on super-normal powers with gusto and secret longings. Either that, or we pooh-pooh it and tell others not to bother with such nonsense that can lead us astray from our *real* spiritual quest. For more on Patanjali's chapter on super-normal powers and his samyama sutras, see the Appendix.

Meanwhile, are we really in a position to judge the existence of super-normal powers, either for or against? It seems that either way we view it, we will be holding ourselves back, because we will be obstructing our true inner nature (whatever it is) with our mental fabrications about such things. Therefore, the best position to take is to have no view at all, continue on the path of purification and opening, and see what happens. If we do that, we will find out the truth of it by and by. It is a scientific approach.

So, in that spirit, we will neither endorse nor debunk super-normal powers here. There is no point in arguing about what we have not experienced for ourselves. Instead, we will be wise to just continue along our path, keeping an open mind for whatever may come. If we focus on the *how* and let the *what* flow naturally from that, we will have much more success with samyama, and all of our practices.

Super-normal powers can be neither possessed nor denied. If and when they occur, they will be a by-product of our practices and spiritual growth, not a cause. Here we are concerned with causes. If we attend to the causes, all the rest will be there.

We already know that samyama brings many practical results in daily life, and therefore has an important role to play in our over all unfoldment. So we can continue with that, not for any particular expression of power we may wish, but for a broad-based opening of our full potential. This is something we can see unfolding in our everyday life over months and years of daily practice.

Some might argue against the practice of samyama itself, suggesting that in the wrong hands it could be misused and cause damage to the practitioner and others. The truth is that it is not possible to use real samyama for ill, other than overdoing and experiencing some excessive inner purification. That is simply too much of a good thing, and can be regulated by prudent self-pacing in practices.

No matter what sutras we are using, no matter how poor our selection, if we are releasing them into inner silence the result will be positive. Negativity cannot flow from pure bliss consciousness. It simply is not possible. This is why we call samyama a *morally self-regulating* practice.

If we do not have enough inner silence present when undertaking samyama, little will happen. If there is inner silence, what happens will be positive. If we *project* a sutra outward, instead of *letting it go* into stillness, with the intention expressing personal power, the strength of the sutra will be greatly diminished. There are some who spend great effort constructing externally projected things, much to their loss of time and progress. It is the building of castles suspended in thin air. It is not samyama. Such activities have nothing to do with spiritual development.

While there are many possibilities for divine expression that can flow from within, the greatest of all these is *Joy*.

Joy is the spontaneous letting go of all that we are into our infinite and eternal nature. It is surrender into that by which all is manifesting. Joy is the essential constituent in all of life and is the greatest siddhi – the greatest of all the super-normal powers. Joy is what has us laughing heartily as we become consciously *One* with the miraculous mystery of life.

The Importance of a Methodical Approach

We have reviewed a variety of expanded applications of the technique of samyama here. While no promises are made about the attainment of so-called *super-normal powers*, the possibility is certainly there. No need to make promises here. We can rely on our own experiences along the path, and find out for ourselves. If we seek promises, better to look to our religious traditions. It is up to us to prove them right or wrong, not by intellectual arguments or by citing the experiences of others. If powers are real, then they will manifest from within us sooner or later. That is what this discussion is about. Speculation is for the idle curious. Let us unfold the real thing, whatever it may be. In the end, we may be pleasantly surprised!

A word of caution should be offered here. We have presented quite a few options to choose from for using samyama in both structured practice and in our daily life. After reading all this, we might feel like the proverbial *kid in a candy store*, not knowing which piece to grab first, and maybe trying to grab all the candy at once. While it has been said here before, and many times throughout all of the AYP writings, still, it cannot be overemphasized that it is best to take on practices one at a time, allowing each one to settle in before taking on another. It can take months or years to assimilate a new practice (not days), depending on our inner matrix of obstructions and the unique course of our purification and opening.

Therefore, it is wise to utilize a methodical approach in undertaking practices, closely monitoring the results each step along the way, and taking subsequent steps in a prudent fashion. This sort of self-paced approach has proven itself to be most fruitful, and an exciting and liberating alternative to the slow spoon-fed methods of the ancient traditions. Clearly, the time for self-directed practice has arrived. In this, it is up to each of us to proceed responsibly on our own path.

If we have a good foundation in deep meditation, or otherwise feel we have abiding inner silence, we may be ready to dip our toe into samyama practice.

However, if we take on sitting samyama practice (as described in Chapter 2) on Monday, dive into cosmic samyama on Tuesday, infuse our asana routine with samyama on Wednesday, and add samyama to all of our prayers on Thursday, we will likely be suffering from a samyama hangover by Friday. Then, on Saturday, our discomfort may force us to drop everything, including the practices we had stabilized before we undertook samyama!

This is obviously not the way to go. There is no way we can shortcut our own process of purification and opening. We can optimize it with effective yoga practices, when soundly applied. But we cannot completely brush aside the natural evolutionary process that needs to unfold within us in its own way. No amount of charging through with discomfort will be more effective than a methodical measured approach.

The effective application of spiritual practices and our journey along the path is a marathon, not a sprint.

In this book on samyama we have gone further in offering multiple angles on practice than we have done with previous practices. We could even say that this book is an open source *do-it-yourself samyama kit*. It is as much a research tool as it is a practice tool. We have both structure and lots of options here.

This approach has been taken because, once inner silence is on the move, it will be expressing in every nook and cranny of our life. If we understand this and are developing the habit of applying the principles of samyama in these multiple expressions of pure bliss consciousness, we will be in a much better position to facilitate them and, hence, the process of our enlightenment.

But none of this is to diminish the importance of structure, and the essential principle of digging the well deeply in one place, instead of digging shallow ineffective holes all over the lot. If spiritual practices are approached in a diluted dabbling way, not much will come of them. It is like that with most things in life, isn't it? We will get out what we put in. In the case of spiritual practices, if we take a methodical, committed approach, we can open the door to abiding inner silence, ecstatic bliss and outpouring divine love. It is worth doing.

So, when we begin a practice, we should commit to it in both structure and implementation over time, subject to adjustments required by prudent self-pacing, as necessary. This means aiming to keep our samyama routine and sutras reasonably stable over time. It is how we will get the best results from them. When we do make additions or modifications, it should be with deliberation, and with the intent to stabilize the change in our routine.

At the same time, it may be appropriate to engage in measured experiments from time to time, and we will no doubt be inspired to do that with the practices in this chapter, and possibly with some of the additional options offered in the Appendix on the *Samyama Sutras of Patanjali*. That is what the presented information is for – methodical evaluation and judicious testing from time to time over the long term. We may also come up with additional approaches of our own. There is nothing wrong with that. The possibilities for improvement in all avenues of life are endless. Spiritual life is no exception.

So maybe we will end up modifying the suggested long term samyama practices that are offered here, and maybe we will not. It is up to us. It is the essence of self-directed practice by responsible seekers of truth. The result will be a continuing evolution of the application of methods that capitalize on the principles of human spiritual transformation. It is about time yoga got on the bandwagon of applied science, yes? It is a good thing.

So let's pursue a methodical approach designed for our systematic purification and opening – optimized by us over time to be progressive, comfortable and safe. And by all means, let's enjoy the ride!

Chapter 4 – Stillness in Action

Since ancient times, it has been known that human spiritual experience includes two components, one that brings great inner peace and forbearance, and another that is ecstatic and dynamic. These two aspects of our nature have been expressed in the mythologies of the many traditions around the world. Whether we subscribe to *Shiva and Shakti, Father God and Holy Spirit*, or any other concepts or icons representing our internal spiritual dynamics, or to no icons other than the neurobiology of enlightenment itself, the inner dynamics will be the same. This is assuming we are actively engaged in effective spiritual practices. It is a matter of cause and effect, determined by the vast and ever-present potential found within every human nervous system. All mythologies and religions spring from this reality. Every human being is a doorway to the divine.

By using the phrase *stillness in action*, we are reducing the dynamic relationship of inner silence and ecstasy to its simplest common denominator. One of them, anyway. We could also say that it is all inner silence, all stillness, all *One*, since even divine ecstasy is swallowed up in *That*. This is the non-dual interpretation of what is happening.

But for now, we will stick with the two components, so we can trace the process occurring in our nervous system as we engage in spiritual practices, and samyama in particular. As we will see, it is all an expression of *Oneness*.

As we consider the implications of *stillness in action*, we will find that there are innumerable aspects involved, and that the essential characteristics of this process are radiance, ecstatic bliss, and unity.

How we participate in all of this is the most remarkable part. We only need to surrender to the divine outpouring, and it reveals its infinite dimensions to us in many aspects of our life. All applications of samyama are for cultivating this natural ability. In fact, all of yoga is for promoting this, thereby freeing us to directly experience our essential nature and full potential in daily living.

Relationship of Inner Silence and Ecstasy

In approaching samyama, inner silence is a prerequisite. Once inner silence is present, samyama practice will lead to its expansion in daily activity, much the way a pump will greatly expand the supply of water once the pump has been primed.

Another prerequisite for samyama is the rise of ecstatic conductivity in the nervous system. Perhaps *prerequisite* is too strong a word for ecstatic conductivity in relation to samyama, because samyama will be effective with inner silence alone, without ecstatic conductivity much in evidence.

As was mentioned earlier, ecstatic conductivity is cultivated with different kinds of practices than are used for the cultivation of inner silence. Inner silence relies almost entirely on the practice of deep meditation, and is then expanded through samyama. Ecstatic conductivity, on the other hand, is cultivated with spinal breathing pranayama, asanas, mudras, bandhas, and tantric sexual methods. These are different classes of practice altogether.

But, interestingly, practices related to the cultivation of ecstatic conductivity enhance both deep meditation and samyama. This is because they loosen the subtle neurobiology. Pranayama is especially effective for this, and the loosening is further facilitated with asanas, mudras, bandhas and tantric methods. These methods that are energy related cultivate the soil of the nervous system to make it a better vehicle for inner silence, or pure bliss consciousness.

So here we have the beginning of the relationship of inner silence and ecstasy. The movement of subtle energy in the body (*prana*), and its unmistakable ecstatic quality, are facilitated by the rise of inner silence. At the same time, the rise of inner silence is facilitated by the movement of inner ecstatic energy. Each enables the other!

Samyama straddles the divide between inner silence and ecstasy, working both sides of the fence, so to speak. As we let go of a sutra into silence, we are stimulating stillness to move. To the extent that we have ecstatic conductivity present, that movement of stillness will take on the quality of ecstasy, while at the same time retaining the quality of bliss, which is an inherent quality of inner silence. The result is moving ecstatic bliss, which is the fuel of divine expression in the world.

Flying on the Wings of Ecstatic Bliss

With the marriage of inner silence and ecstasy, a new dynamic is born. We could call it *ecstatic bliss*, but that hardly explains it. We sometimes use the phrase *abiding inner silence, ecstatic bliss and outpouring divine love*. This more fully captures the dynamic that is occurring. There is stillness – *abiding inner silence*. There is an inner radiance that contains the qualities of both pure bliss consciousness and ecstatic conductivity – *ecstatic bliss*. And there is movement outward as the flow of radiance seeks to express itself through the nervous system – *outpouring divine love*.

From the point of view of the practitioner, we find a lot of pleasure in this on many levels. It is physical and psychological pleasure. The outflowing is luminous and the world becomes luminous as well. Not that the nature of the world has changed, but we have changed in the way we see it. We see it for what it really is – an infinite flow of energy that is in a constant joyous dance. The negative interpretations that predominate in so much of human life are seen in an entirely different light. The foibles of mind are seen to be outrageous!

So what do we do when we come to see the world in this way? Do we run away and hide out in a cave? No way. Surely there are ways to help everyone to see what we see. From within ourselves we are moved to do that – to help in whatever way we can. It is an outpouring, an outpouring of divine love.

This third element, the outpouring, that comes from the merging of our inner silence and ecstatic conductivity is the proverbial child of enlightenment. It has been called Christ, Jivan Mukti, savior. It is not we in the personal egoic sense who become this. It is the divine flowing through us that is this birth, this outpouring, and we become consciously dissolved in *It*, surrendered to *It*.

Samyama plays an important role in cultivating and stabilizing this divine flow. As we have discussed here again and again, the essence of samyama is surrender, letting go. If we set up the initial conditions of inner silence and ecstatic conductivity with our other practices, and then engage in daily samyama practice, the merging and divine birth will occur.

Then we will find ourselves flying on the wings of ecstatic bliss in everything we do. And we will be surrounded by wonderful miraculous happenings. All of nature rushes to support a divine outpouring once it has begun. Once the divine pump has been primed, the flow increases without limit. By learning to let go we are able to unleash infinite good in the world.

Let Go and Let God

Why would any of us choose this, the union of our personal self with something so vast and powerful within us? One simple reason – *happiness*.

We have a powerful instinct that is part of our nature, which is always seeking our ultimate happiness. We may not know what that happiness is, or exactly how to go about finding it, but the urge is there in all of us. If it were not, we would have no motivation to do anything in this world. All that we do is driven by the singular need to be happy. We are wired that way since birth, and probably long before. We have been born here to discover it in ourselves.

It is for this that we travel the globe far and wide and seek to accumulate all that we can in the hope of finding happiness. We have even gone into outer space to seek it. Yet, the more we attain and acquire, the greater the mystery grows, because there is no end to the external seeking.

It is a great paradox that our outer happiness ultimately depends on an inner journey. Only when we are taking the inner journey can we begin to function in the outer world with a sense of fulfillment. Our freedom and happiness are not *out there*. They are *in here*.

Does this mean we should shun the world and focus exclusively on the inner life? Ironically shunning the world is as much an external projection of our seeking for happiness as traveling far and wide is. Why? Because there is a double paradox here. While it is true that we can only find our happiness by going within, it is equally true that once we are going within, our happiness will only be found in the outer world. This is why we say the fruit of yoga practices will not be found within the practices themselves, but in our daily activities. It is by *living* that we find the divine in life. It is in our external surroundings where we will finally find ourselves. By unfolding from within we can accomplish this.

The truth is, it does not matter if we are living in a cave in a remote region, or in the middle of a busy city. If we are engaged in effective spiritual practices on a daily basis and going out and being active in the world in some way, we will be progressing equally well. Beyond the dynamic of daily practices and keeping active in-between practice sessions, the primary factor will be the matrix of obstructions within us that we are dissolving. This we can manage ably within the context of our practices and lifestyle, with the prudent application of the principles of self-pacing. If we are clear about what we are doing, and following our course with persistence over the long term, we will achieve the desired result. Our external environment will not matter in this. Everything is an expression of the same *Oneness* we are unfolding.

While we can mention a thousand reasons why we find ourselves delayed in taking on a structured daily routine of effective spiritual practices, there is really only one thing that is necessary to make it happen – *active surrender*. By active surrender, we mean a combination of intense desire and a willingness to work within whatever situation we may find ourselves.

We can be sure that if we are putting in the time twice daily, we will have the results in time. If we do what is necessary, and let go, all things will come to us. It is the essence of samyama – picking up the object of our desire and letting it go, again and again. It is by this process, in practices and in life, that lasting happiness is finally found.

Liberation is not a striving. It is returning to our intention, letting go, and allowing the flow, doing that again and again for as long as it takes. It is the constant act of intention, expanding through the ongoing experience of ... *Let go and let God.*

Appendix

The Samyama Sutras of Patanjali

We owe a great debt to the ancient sage, Patanjali, for documenting the practices and experiences of yoga as he saw them. His *Yoga Sutras* are an important benchmark on the methods of human spiritual transformation, and have been guiding practitioners for centuries.

The *Yoga Sutras* are a concise document, comprised of four chapters. Numerous translations into many languages from the original Sanskrit are readily available in books and on the Internet. Some of these can be found on the *Links Page* of the AYP website (see website address at the end of this book).

The third chapter of the *Yoga Sutras* is devoted to samyama and *super-normal powers*, and offers a series of 30 sutras that can be used. More importantly, these sutras are offered within the context of the journey to enlightenment, not only from the point of view of samyama practice, but in relation to the rest of yoga. In other words, super-normal powers are not really about super-normal powers. They are about the over all enlightenment journey, and all that it entails in the realms of practice and experience. Without this context, considering super-normal powers amounts to little more than fanciful dabbling, and not much will come out of it. We have all been there, and that is why some of us are still slogging along the path instead of dancing in the light. Maybe we are doing some of both. It is a good sign!

As has been mentioned again and again in this book, inner silence is the essential prerequisite for successful samyama practice. And the rise of ecstatic conductivity is an important concurrent support. Both of these aspects of our nature are cultivated using other means on the eight-limbed tree of yoga, with deep meditation and spinal breathing pranayama being chief among these. If we have done this before embarking on our samyama practice, the results will be there, and they will be *morally self-regulating* besides. This means that we will find more benefit from samyama, while not being caught up in either the anticipation or the results. This fulfills Patanjali's exhortation not to confuse the scenery for the goal, no matter how glorious or inviting the prospects for experience may be. It is good common sense.

From the AYP point of view, we always favor the practice over the *sirens* of spiritual experience. No matter what the sutra and its corresponding siddhi may be, samyama practice is always about purification and opening, and not about running off into fanciful adventures in our favorite celestial realm. Experiences do not produce spiritual progress. Practices do.

It is in that spirit that we present Patanjali's samyama sutras in a practical way that can be used for research by serious practitioners moving forward along the road of applied yoga science.

This is not intended to be a scholarly analysis of the *Samyama Sutras of Patanjali*. Plenty of those are available for the asking. Rather, English translations have been used to condense Patanjali's samyama sutras into a series of simple, useable code words and phrases that can be used for research in practice by those who are so inclined. The sutras presented here are interpretations, and should be regarded as such.

The practitioner should feel free to question the effectiveness and credibility of Patanjali's samyama sutras themselves, whether in original or interpreted form. When things have been written down and passed on for centuries, there is tendency to take their validity for granted. Certainly, written truths last, but we must also be able to verify them. Without verification, whatever we are reading is only a proposition. That applies to the centuries-old writing of Patanjali, or anything that is being written now on these matters, including this book! It is reliable causes and effects we are seeking for the purpose of promoting human spiritual transformation. If we approach all teachings from that perspective, we will be in a position to reap the most from them, and ultimately manifest the truth from within our own nervous system, which is where all yoga comes from.

Research for well-established Practitioners

It is recommended that research with the sutras listed here not be attempted until the samyama routines provided in Chapters 2 and 3 have been undertaken and stabilized in daily practice. This is not because there is anything untoward or dangerous in this Appendix. It is a practical matter. Samyama is only effective when undertaken using a stable series of sutras on a daily basis over time. Therefore, as has been pointed out already in the book, a methodical approach will serve our needs much better than jumping around and trying many different things, only to end up with nothing.

For that reason, consider this Appendix to be something for later. Maybe much later. Or maybe never. After all, considerable effort has gone into constructing the samyama routines earlier in this book. There is no need to reinvent the wheel, assuming that it has been reasonably well-invented so far. That is for each practitioner to decide for themselves.

This Appendix is provided for further exploration, once a stable samyama routine has been established.

These samyama sutras have been interpreted and condensed by the author. In some cases, alternative interpretations are possible, and they may be adjusted if it is felt to be necessary. They may also be translated to the practitioner's first language. If there are any doubts, going back and reviewing the *Yoga Sutras of Patanjali* is suggested.

Regarding the sutras as presented, and their possible use, some clarifications should be mentioned.

In some cases there is redundancy in the expression with the word *inner* included in the sutra itself. By redundancy, it is meant that samyama is merging an object (the sutra) with inner silence, or pure bliss consciousness. In Patanjali's sutras the element of inner silence is sometimes included in the sutra itself. It can be expressed as purusha, transcendence, stillness, *inner*, or other words or phrases. For our purposes, we have minimized the use of such designations in the previous chapters. In the main AYP sutra list in Chapter 2, the word *inner* is used only in relation to *inner sensuality*, where it was felt an emphasis on transcendence would be helpful for developing pratyahara (introversion of sense perception, while dissolving attachment). In all of the other sutras, the actuality of *inner* is included in the technique of samyama itself. So, when we do samyama with the sutra *strength*, for example, this is radiating strength from within inner silence by virtue of the process of samyama. It is the same with most of the sutras on the AYP list. In the case of interpreting the *Samyama Sutras of Patanjali*, the redundancy (including *inner* in the sutra) is retained so as not to depart from the original more than we have already. So you find the word *inner* (meaning *transcendent,* etc.) in several of the sutras.

Another variation is found in the use of the Sanskrit word *Akasha*, which means *inner space*. It is the only Sanskrit word retained in the list of Patanjali's samyama sutras. It is also the only Sanskrit word in the AYP sutra list, used in *Akasha – Lightness of Air*. In the Patanjali list, it is also found in relation to the senses (hearing, etc.). In truth, *Inner Space* can replace the word *Akasha* in any sutra where it is found, with equal effectiveness (it is used this way in the *Secrets of Wilder* novel in the lightness sutra). For effective samyama, it is not a matter of having the right word. It is a matter of the sutra having a clear meaning for us. This is why translation of sutras to our most familiar language is acceptable. The more familiar the language, the more familiar the meaning of the sutra (code word) when released into inner silence.

Of course, with a mantra we use for deep meditation, this is not the case. Mantras are not used for meaning, but for inner sound quality in our nervous system, and we do not translate a mantra to another language because, in the way it is being used in deep meditation, it has no meaning. But for sutras used in samyama, we are using the meanings, so this involves language and condensing ideas into as few words as possible, so they can be easily let go into stillness, carrying their meaning with them into the infinite realm of pure bliss consciousness. And then we have the result radiating out from that…

It is suggested that, if any of the Patanjali samyama sutras are explored, they be explored one at a time within the context of our well-established sitting samyama routine.

So, say we'd like to experiment with a sutra to increase calmness in our life. In that case, we could add *bronchial tube* to our sutra list for several sessions and see what comes out of it. By experimenting with one sutra at a time in our already stable routine of samyama, any effects will be more easily noticed and associated with the addition of the individual sutra. If we add on two or more sutras, it will be difficult to know what is doing what, and also difficult to sustain a stable practice, especially if we are adding on and taking off multiple sutras. Remember, it is very important to be methodical in samyama practice.

So, with that, take a look at the following interpretations of Patanjali's samyama sutras. The sutras are presented in **bold type**, followed by a hyphen and a brief description of the predicted result. They are given in the same order they are listed in the *Yoga Sutras of Patanjali*. Remember to maintain a stable daily practice, prudently applying the principles of self-pacing, as needed, and enjoy!

1. **Past, Present, Future** – knowledge of the past and the future.

2. **Word, Object, Idea** – knowledge of the meaning of the sounds produced by all beings.

3. **Latent Impressions** – knowledge of previous births.

4. **Notions of (insert person's name)** – knowledge of the person's mind.

5. **Body's Appearance** – disappearance of the body from view.

6. **Karma** – foreknowledge of death.

7. **Friendliness** – increased friendliness.

8. **Strength** – increased strength.

9. **Inner Light on (insert name of object, person or place)** – knowledge of the object, person, or place obstructed from view or at a great distance.

10. **Sun** – knowledge of the cosmic regions.

11. **Moon** – knowledge of the arrangement of the stars.

12. **Pole Star** – knowledge of the motions of the stars.

13. **Navel** – knowledge of the composition of the body.

14. **Trachea** – subduing hunger and thirst.

15. **Bronchial Tube** – calmness.

16. **Coronal Light of (insert name of deity, higher being, or class of beings - siddhas, devas, angels, fairies, etc.)** – vision of the deity, higher being, or class of beings.

17. **Inner Intuition** – omniscience.

18. **Heart** – knowledge of the mind.

19. **Inner Sensuality** – refined sensory ability (all five senses), and transcendence of attachment to sensory experience (pratyahara).

20. **Bondage of the Mind** – knowledge of occupying another body.

21. **Breath** – immunity from disruptions in the external physical environment, and exit from the body at will.

22. **Digestion** – radiance of the body from inside.

23. **Akasha Hearing** – divine sense of hearing. Can also be applied to touch, sight, taste and smell. For enhancement of the individual senses.

24. **Akasha - Lightness of Air** – lightness of the body and passage through the air.

25. **Unseen Obstructions** – removal of unknown veils covering illumination.

26. **Elements** – mastery over the five elements (earth, water, fire, air, and inner space), enabling manipulation of all matter, including the size, appearance and condition of the body.

27. **Organs of Action** – mastery over the five organs of action (hands, feet, vocal chords, sexual organ and root/anus) and the ability to project actions from a distance.

28. **Inner Intellect** – stewardship of all beings.

29. **Renunciation** – destruction of the seeds of illusion, yielding liberation.

30. **Sequence of Moments** – ability to differentiate self from illusion.

Further Reading and Support

Yogani is an American spiritual scientist who, for more than thirty years, has been integrating ancient techniques from around the world which cultivate human spiritual transformation. The approach he has developed is non-sectarian, and open to all. In the order published, his books include:

Advanced Yoga Practices – Easy Lessons for Ecstatic Living
A large user-friendly textbook providing 240 detailed lessons on the AYP integrated system of yoga practices.

The Secrets of Wilder – A Novel
The story of young Americans discovering and utilizing actual secret practices leading to human spiritual transformation.

The AYP Enlightenment Series
Easy-to-read instruction books on yoga practices, including:

- *Deep Meditation – Pathway to Personal Freedom*
- *Spinal Breathing Pranayama – Journey to Inner Space*
- *Tantra – Discovering the Power of Pre-Orgasmic Sex*
- *Asanas, Mudras and Bandhas – Awakening Ecstatic Kundalini*
- *Samyama – Cultivating Stillness in Action, Siddhis and Miracles*
- *Diet, Shatkarmas and Amaroli – Yogic Nutrition and Cleansing for Health and Spirit* (1st half 2007)
- *Self Inquiry – Dawn of the Witness and the End of Suffering* (1st half 2007)
- *Bhakti and Karma Yoga – The Science of Devotion and Liberation Through Action* (2nd half 2007)
- *Eight Limbs of Yoga – The Structure and Pacing of Self-Directed Spiritual Practice* (2nd half 2007)

For up-to-date information on the writings of Yogani, and for the free *AYP Support Forums*, please visit:

www.advancedyogapractices.com

CPSIA information can be obtained at www.ICGtesting.com
Printed in the USA
BVOW07s2356190813

328940BV00001B/19/A